Deeper Still

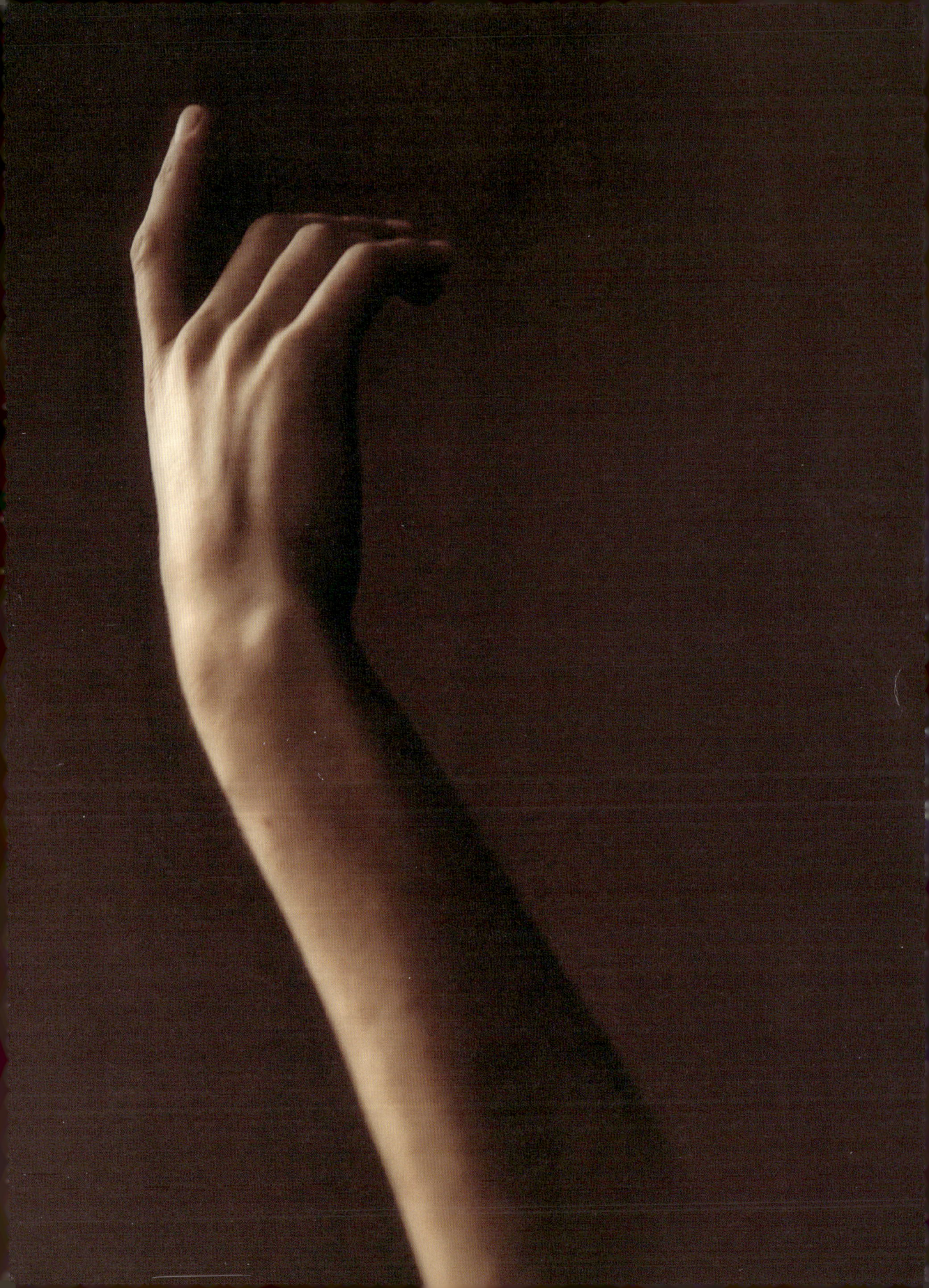

Deeper Still

Authentic embodiment for yoga teachers

John Stirk

Foreword
Carol Nelson

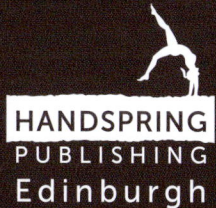

HANDSPRING
PUBLISHING
Edinburgh

HANDSPRING PUBLISHING LIMITED
The Old Manse, Fountainhall,
Pencaitland, East Lothian
EH34 5EY, Scotland
Tel: +44 1875 341 859
Website: www.handspringpublishing.com

First published 2021 in the United Kingdom by Handspring Publishing Limited

Copyright ©Handspring Publishing Limited 2021

The three photographs in Chapter 5 on pages 69 and 74 are reproduced with kind permission from Guimberteau J.-C. (2015) Architecture of Living Fascia, Edinburgh: Handspring Publishing Limited (from page 24, Figure 1.14 and Figure 3.6B). All other photographs are by Sarah Stirk.

All rights reserved. No parts of this publication may be reproduced or transmitted in any form or by any means, electronic or mechanical, including photocopying, recording, or any information storage and retrieval system, without either the prior written permission of the publisher or a license permitting restricted copying in the United Kingdom issued by the Copyright Licensing Agency Ltd, Saffron House, 6-10 Kirby Street, London EC1N 8TS.

The rights of John Stirk to be identified as the Author of this text have been asserted in accordance with the Copyright, Designs and Patents Acts 1988.

ISBN 978-1-912085-71-2
ISBN (Kindle eBook) 978-1-912085-72-9

British Library Cataloguing in Publication Data
A catalogue record for this book is available from the British Library

Library of Congress Cataloguing in Publication Data
A catalog record for this book is available from the Library of Congress

Notice
Neither the Publisher nor the Author assumes any responsibility for any loss or injury and/or damage to persons or property arising out of or relating to any use of the material contained in this book. It is the responsibility of the treating practitioner, relying on independent expertise and knowledge of the patient, to determine the best treatment and method of application for the patient.

Commissioning Editor Sarena Wolfaard
Project Manager Morven Dean
Copy Editor Sally Davies
Cover and Design Direction Bruce Hogarth
Indexer Aptara, India
Typesetter DSM, India
Printer Bell and Bain, UK

Cover image Sarah Stirk

The Publisher's policy is to use paper manufactured from sustainable forests

Contents

Foreword by Carol Nelson — vii
About the Author — ix
Acknowledgments — x
Prologue — xi
Introduction — xx

1. The Reality — 1
2. Process — 13
3. Embodiment — 25
4. Dividing the indivisible — 35
5. Sensing — 61
6. Fields — 83
7. Minds and hearts — 109
8. Insight and wisdom — 125
9. Authentic teaching — 139
10. Unification — 151

References — 183
Index — 185

Dedication

To Hannah for her love and wisdom

FOREWORD *by* Carol Nelson

It was an unusually balmy and blustery November evening in 1990 when John Stirk quite literally blew into my yoga studio in Brookline, Massachusetts. The weather was not the only unusual aspect of that evening. He was a force – scrolls under his arms filled with stick figures and arrows, hoping to point us in a new direction. His enthusiasm was matched only by his desire to communicate his process and understanding of the essence of yoga.

He was masterful, articulate and there was something uniquely different about his approach. He has been our guide, our mentor, and even, occasionally, our entertainer ever since. He has taught us to search within our very beings, and to be deeply enriched by this endeavor, free from techniques, systems, or ideals.

My yoga career began in the 1970s when I first met and studied with B. K. S. Iyengar. Since that time, I have observed the trajectory of yoga evolve from a relatively obscure unknown to a household word with millions of people "doing" something called yoga.

The physical aspect of yoga is a beautiful point of entry. It is important and remains a connecting thread throughout. However, to reduce yoga to an act of physical prowess, a fitness commodity, or even an advertising gimmick misses the profound depth and beauty of this art.

Yoga needs to reclaim its ancient role – to remind us of what we could be, of what unites us, of our common humanity. *Deeper Still* invites us to explore this paradigm shift. Yoga becomes a lens through which we find meaning within ourselves. With his insight and wisdom John Stirk guides us towards the unifying spirit found within the quiet inner spaces of our own hearts and minds.

Deeper Still is a groundbreaking body of work and one of the most original I have ever encountered. Uniquely John, yet his ideas are substantiated by modern philosophical and psychological thought, ancient wisdom teachings, and even quantum science. I believe this work lies on the frontier of the evolution of yoga practice and teaching. It is complex in its scope and depth. The subject demands it.

It is for the skilled specialist, mature (in age and number of years practicing) meditator, yogi. It is a gift to the yoga community ready and eager to go beyond the basics of mechanics and enter into the more advanced expressions of the science of yoga, the nature of mind and consciousness, and how these expressions relate to our purpose, our humanity, and what unites us.

For nearly 30 consecutive years, John Stirk has come to Brookline or Martha's Vineyard, MA, to share his unique teachings with us. We have emerged, from all over the

FOREWORD *by* Carol Nelson *continued*

country, as a family, traveling together on a journey to yoga. He has taken us on undiscovered paths that awaken our senses and consciousness to new and untapped possibility and potential. *Deeper Still* brings to the reader the felt quality of experience and discovery that one finds in his classes.

There are no levels separating beginners from advanced students in John Stirk's classes. There are no advanced certificates of completion either. What you do find is an authentic embodiment to Presence.

Carol Nelson BA
Founder Director Creative Yoga Studio, Brookline, MA, USA
The Salon for Creative Yoga, Martha's Vineyard, MA, USA
www.yogaonmv.com
November 2020

About the Author

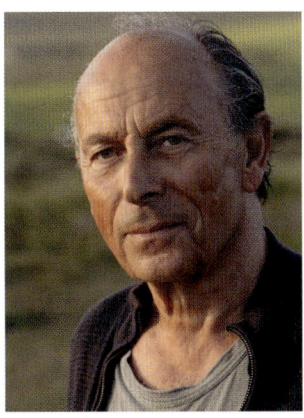

John Stirk is a yoga teacher and author with a background in osteopathy. He has been teaching yoga since 1974. He graduated as an osteopath in 1983 from the College of Osteopaths in London where he subsequently lectured in biomechanics and practical osteopathy. He was made a fellow of the college in 1995. His association with R. D. Laing in the 1970s and 1980s and his attraction to the teaching of J. Krishnamurti have inspired his approach to a quality of consciousness realized through hatha yoga practices.

John stopped practicing osteopathy in 2005 to focus exclusively on yoga teaching and use his osteopathic and philosophical understanding to inform teachers. His approach has influenced many teachers in the UK and internationally.

His interests lie in the power of group work and the potential insight and wisdom that arise spontaneously within the group field. He invites yoga teachers to take a step further: to trust and share their own insight and wisdom with their students by using physical sensitivity as a springboard to an alternative consciousness.

John is the author of several books, notably *The Original Body: Primal Movement for Yoga Teachers* (Handspring 2015). He teaches in the UK and internationally and conducts courses for teachers, including the highly successful "What Lies Beneath" course.

John is based in London and East Sussex where he lives with his wife Lolly Stirk, who is a childbirth activist, pioneer of yoga for pregnancy, and founder member of the Active Birth Movement and Yoga Birth. Their daughter Sarah created the photographic images for this book.

Acknowledgments

I would like to thank: my daughter Sarah Stirk for the photographs in this book and for her constructive observations throughout what has been an inspired and special collaboration; yoga teacher Paula Andreewitch for allowing us to capture her practice; my long-term students for their continued willingness to practice with me and for their inspiring feedback; my soulmate Lolly for her continued support, constructive advice and observations and the endless discussions over many years on the nature of everything; Carol and Paul Marks Stopforth in Boston for their willingness to discuss *Deeper Still* on a regular basis; Barry and Sheila Hay-Gordon for supporting me in ways they may not be aware of; American yogini and friend Carol Nelson in Martha's Vineyard for her wisdom and friendship; Jonathan Sattin, Founder and Managing Director Triyoga London, for his continued support and friendship; and Sarena Wolfaard at Handspring, for further engaging with me on this book, and her talented team for their guidance with the production.

John Stirk
East Dean, UK
October 2020

Prologue

The pigeon

The basement toilet of the Hyde Park salon had a small window looking out onto the well of the building. I sat head in hands. The marijuana proffered by a junior member of staff had given me stomach cramps. The business was failing and I had a new family. Feeling dizzy and hopeless I bent forward chest to knees. My mind lit up, I felt a deep connection between my thighs and lower back. I moved backward and forward several times, challenging the reality of the sensations. The light in my mind grew brighter. A scruffy London pigeon sat on the ledge of the open window just above my head. I looked at it and said: *I'm going to be a Yoga teacher*. It squawked its approval. It was 1974.

Lolly

There had to be something more than the King's Road, Chelsea. I had no idea what *more* was until I met Lolly. She came into the salon, a beautiful hippy girl. The people Lolly introduced me to were looking at the nature of consciousness, the complexity of relationships, what went on within and between us, and what lay beneath our conditioning. I had come home. On our wedding day a friend of a friend gifted a book, *Life Ahead*, by someone called Krishnamurti. Published in 1963 it was addressed to young people. I did not read it until some years later.

Three life-changing things happened to me in 1973. I met and fell in love with Lolly. I became a part of her extraordinary group and I discovered yoga. My education had begun. Given the confidence by her yoga practice, Lolly decided to give birth to Sarah at home. On October 10th, 1974, the fourth life-changing thing happened – a beautiful and wise baby girl.

Lolly and several of the group had opened one of the first vegetarian restaurants in London, Wheat, which was close to Abbey Road Studios. Many famous musicians as well as artists, actors, and psychotherapists came. Wheat was a hub of creative and intellectual discourse and the food was great. Due to bad posture and a riding accident, I had had increasingly severe back pain for some years. Lolly set to work. She had learnt yoga from Iyengar and his student Dona Holleman and was my first teacher. The effect of a few basic poses was immediate and transformative. Within a few weeks the pain went. I could think clearly. I discovered my mind! The first few months of intense practice brought on night sweats. As a child I had had a recurring nightmare that I had forgotten. It returned, released, and never came back. I realized the potential of this work and began teaching a few small groups how to stretch.

Another kind of group

The seventies were the *aha* years. Transformative experiences were common. The group was breathtakingly progressive. It was a radical beginning: stretching inspired by Iyengar combined with a close look at the depth, range, potential, and fragility of the mind. The group was comprised of psychotherapists, yoga teachers, bodyworkers, writers, and artists. The anthropologist Francis Huxley, nephew of Aldous, made a valuable contribution.

Ronnie

I had not heard of R. D. Laing. His name would frequently come up. "Ronnie says this," "Ronnie says that." Who was this person? On meeting him I was struck by his depth of presence. The therapist's measured silences perhaps! But there was something else: a deep and broad *knowing* I had not encountered before. He appeared to know more about the mind and *experience* than anyone at that time. His books were a global success, yet you could learn as much about yourself by being in the same room. He had the extraordinary gift of being able to enter the world of psychotic individuals. This was something he carried with him, an uncanny affinity with other minds, intended or not. "*When I started to meet psychotic patients professionally, I found to my alarm that sometimes I could see their point of view only too well*" (Clay 1996). Laing was cutting edge and courageous. His books and growing reputation for "understanding madness" highlighted the shortcomings of the psychiatry of the day. His capacity for *being* underscored his skill for listening and *seeing*. Ronnie was a *seer*. There are numerous accounts of his insight into the minds of severely disturbed people. He was a teacher without teaching, just with time spent, one way or the other. I read his books. R. D. Laing's Glaswegian common sense resonated ("*just get on with it*"). I was raised by my grandmother Hannah and subject to ongoing Jewish wisdom. Hannah had lost a son to glandular fever and when, as a baby, I was made a ward of court due to my parents' separation I was a welcome replacement. If we are going to be grounded, be grounded in common sense.

The group stretched, discussed, read, and gathered around R. D. We dug deeply, defying the norm in an attempt to free ourselves and *see* our conditioned patterns. The parties and meetings were often cut from the same cloth. The social aspect and quest for realization were indivisible. We sang. Ronnie played piano: Cole Porter, Gershwin. We danced as our kids ranged between us. The focus was the moment, any moment, this moment any time and place. A deep awareness prevailed regardless of the setting. Ronnie's affinity with the mind dripped down into the group.

Plenty to draw from

There was plenty to draw from. In the frame were Krishnamurti, Wilhelm Reich, Alexander Lowen, Rajneesh, Iyengar, Matthias Alexander, Moshe Feldenkrais, Ram Dass, and others. Fritjof Capra was feted for his book *The Tao of Physics*. People were reading Arthur Janov's *The Primal Scream* and getting their jaws worked on. Rajneesh had a center just off the Edgware Road in West London. Devotees were "whooing" and jumping, and getting it out at Sufi-type workshops. Frédérick Leboyer was advocating putting babies in a tub of warm water on delivery to gently welcome them into the world. Michel Odent was pioneering birth *in* water in Pithiviers, France. R. D. Laing had organized (safe) houses around London (The Philadelphia Association), where disturbed people could see therapists and were given the space they needed to heal without medication. Several yoga teachers in the group taught at the houses.

There were few yoga centers in London in the early to mid-seventies. Teachers used community halls, private homes, and any space fit for purpose. Iyengar would come. I saw him twice, once observing him teach a class and again at the reinauguration of the

Maida Vale Iyengar centre in 1984. It was packed. He spoke at length answering questions, pointing out that he had taught the *jumping*s (Ashtanga) back in 1962, adding: *"But what happens in the jump – in the jump you are out of your body!"*

A band of stretchers

We went ahead and stretched. I had no training, but the Iyengar flavor was in the background. I gleaned some relevant anatomy and read about yoga. The group was made up of the psychotherapists and those of us who were body-focused. There were four of us, a band of stretchers: Arthur Balaskas, Peter Walker, Jonathan Shaw, and myself. We stretched ourselves, stretched each other, and stretched other people. We were prolific. Over the next few years Arthur published *Body Life*. I published my first book with Arthur: *Soft Exercise: The Complete Book of Stretching*. Peter published *Going for Gold* with Daley Thompson on stretching for athletes and later pioneered baby massage, publishing several books. Peter is still going strong, writing and teaching internationally. Jonathan had developed the knack of articulating the entire body through the limbs with extraordinary effect. He moved to Amsterdam where he developed a large following.

We met several times a week and came up with techniques. If it moved, stretch it. If it didn't move, stretch it until it did move. We discussed ideas on how bodywork might help the human condition. There were plenty of themes coming out of Esalen, California, but we stayed with the stretching, feeling that reliance on a practitioner, although a helpful adjunct, did not have the same impact as the work we could do for ourselves. I still have this philosophy while being well aware of the value of treatment when necessary.

We favored the Western approach to the body–mind, each one of us developing a personal library. Among the most useful books were Wilhelm Reich's *Character Analysis* and *The Function of The Orgasm* and Alexander Lowen's *Language of the Body*. Their slant on body armoring and emotional health was and still is pertinent. We sought the anatomy and physiology that supported our practice. There was little reference to fascia in those days. Ida Rolf published her seminal book on Rolfing in 1977. I read the Krishnamurti book. I have since read all his books plus several on his life. I am still taken by his clarity and directness. His expectations are demanding and elusive, and his message is extraordinary and essential.

Ronnie remained in the background or foreground for some time, recommending books and sharing insight. At one point he organized *rebirthing* workshops. This was not the rebirthing of one-to-one breathwork. The "unborn" would adopt a fetal position within a tunnel of six to eight people simulating a womb. The idea was to "get out" through a small space (the pelvic floor) in the tunnel. You were unlucky (or lucky, depending on subconscious needs) if you had a womb determined to make you work. Pushing with the feet, straightening the knees, and negotiating the head and shoulders were exhausting. We took it on the road. A large community hall portrayed emotional devastation, men sobbing for their mothers, as they rested their heads on the chests of caring women.

Lolly, meantime, was pioneering a radical approach to preparation for labour and birth. Giving birth to Sarah at home and having used yoga as the preparation inspired her to help women in the same way. Women in the group were changing policies on birth, encouraging women to take back control of their bodies. Lolly was a founder member of the Active Birth Movement with Janet Balaskas and part of the team that organized the "Birthrights Rally" on Hampstead Heath in 1984. Lolly remains a leading light in the birth world, gives workshops for pregnant women and their partners in the UK, and continues to train teachers in her work in the UK and internationally.

The Green Room

We stretched through the seventies into the early eighties. We set up a room in our home – the "Green Room" – where Lolly held the first pregnancy and postnatal yoga classes in London and I worked with a few groups of four or five. Occasionally during an evening session, the door would quietly open and Sarah at five years old would enter in her pyjamas, look around, choose someone (in child pose!) and apply her body weight through her hand onto their sacrum. She would move around the room making adjustments and once satisfied leave as quietly as she had arrived. It added to the magic of the sessions. Sarah is now an accomplished photographer. I am privileged to have her images in this book.

Clients would lie backward over a wooden bench, with a folded blanket for comfort. I would take their arms and open their chests. People came back. I was busy. I had no formal training. My practice was based on subjective experience, a growing understanding of the need for sensitivity, and the information I gleaned from various sources.

My clients included a young Stephen Russell. He came for regular sessions and we became friends. Some years later he published *Urban Warrior* under the name of Barefoot Doctor, a book that projected him into the public eye. We have often met over many years. Sadly, Steve passed on recently. I will miss him. At a time when the Green Room was in-operative, I rented a space above a French restaurant in Little Venice. Jonathan Satin, a lawyer, came to be stretched. He would come from the office. At the end of the initial sessions his shirt would be stained brown as he sweated out his coffee and nicotine habit. This soon passed. Jonathan gave up coffee and cigarettes and, after working with me for a number of years, took up meditation. In the year 2000 he opened his first triyoga studio in Primrose Hill. It was and is highly successful, with five centers throughout London. We remain friends and I enjoy running workshops at the Camden studio.

Osteopathy

I wanted to know more and osteopathy seemed the obvious choice. In 1983 I enrolled with the College of Osteopaths, one of the few schools of its kind at the time. The College offered mature students an osteopathic training spread over five years. Students without funding or a grant could study while continuing to earn a living.

In my first year, having been shown some basic soft tissue techniques, impatience and enthusiasm prompted me to ask the Dean of the College, Joseph Goodman (Joe), who also practiced naturopathy and acupuncture, if I could work a day or two a week in his busy clinics. He would send me in, a first-year osteopathic student, green at the gills, cubicle after cubicle. This is what I had asked for and was the experience I needed.

Joe chose the patients who were OK for me to work on, and there were many. At first my hands would ache and then they began to tingle and heat up. The healer was stirring. At first I was only allowed to work on feet. One long, hot summer I spent two days every week on sweaty, sometimes odorous, and occasionally pleasant feet. Feet belonging to people with a diversity of problems passed through my hands. I graduated to legs, shoulders, and eventually lower backs. Patients would ask for me by name, they would talk about their issues, and I was happy to listen. Time spent with the group and Ronnie Laing had given me an insight into therapy. This aside, I was attentive. Empathy and hands-on worked wonders. I stayed at Joe's practice for three years and am grateful to him to this day. Yoga was teaching me about my body and mind. I now had hands!

In 1983 I had published a book on stretching, *Soft Exercise,* and had a reputation as a "stretching–yoga teacher," travelling around and giving workshops. I would run classes here and there while studying osteopathy and working for Joe. Stretching classes and one-to-ones continued, and now I was adding soft tissue work and articulatory techniques.

People with pain would come and responded well. I graduated as an osteopath in 1988 and published *Structural Fitness* that year.

The enriching experience of "getting people better" took over from the classes. I cut down to one weekly class. By the time I graduated as an osteopath I had a busy practice in the flat in Maida Vale. I focused mainly on the osteopathic practice but continued with a few one-to-one stretching sessions, and would sometimes incorporate both in a session. Osteopathy took center stage. I articulated, massaged, and occasionally applied a high velocity thrust (HVT), which I later abandoned. Although effective, HVTs could be traumatic. There were other ways to release the tension of painful episodes. Working on my own body prepared me for osteopathic practice in an unexpected way. I could sense into other people's bodies through the awakening sensory experience of my own body (the sensory field). I had additional insight into what others were feeling. As I treated an area, the same area would awaken in my own body: spine to spine, hip to hip, shoulder to shoulder, and so on. I learnt a lot from teaching practical osteopathy at the College, became a part of the team who ran the College, and was made a Fellow in 1995.

At Joe's I had been put in at the deep end, was *learning on my feet,* and had developed an effective way of working tissue. I favored an approach used by Rolfers before I developed my own approach. It involved a slow hooking into the tissue, waiting for the spread to come, and making space in the body. It is a fact highlighted by all bodyworkers – that surface work influences the entire body.

I learnt about people's pain, the varying texture of tissue, and received first-hand confirmation of the extent to which emotion is held by the body. I did not know why so many clients improved so quickly, but they did, often dramatically.

Although technique provided a basis, clients' variability responded well to a certain quality of listening. The involuntary aspects of the body worked their way in with my increasing interest in cranial osteopathy stemming from Sutherland's pioneering work and John Upledger's inspired Craniosacral Therapy (CST). I loved working with babies. One finger on a soft pulsatile sacrum and perhaps one over the solar plexus had the desired effect. Mothers reported their babies would sometimes scream on the way home and then for the first time sleep for seven or eight hours. It is the same kind of magic that is felt in class work – the magic of no expectation, of understating. We can treat ourselves and others like babies.

The osteopath and the yoga teacher

Osteopathy gave me a level of knowledge of anatomy, physiology, and biomechanics I could not have found elsewhere. Osteopathic practice taught me about a variety of acute and chronic conditions, how to spot them, and whether someone would be safe in class work. It confirmed that no two bodies, minds, or personal histories are alike. Yoga has taught me the importance of working on oneself. Many students who came to class work no longer needed treatment, and if they did needed it less frequently. There are crossovers between osteopathic practice and teaching yoga. Yoga and osteopathy inform each other.

Osteopaths and yoga teachers:

- can see into the bodies of others, visualize how they are organized: the osteopath from outside in, the yoga teacher from inside out

- are aware of the emotional investment in physical holding patterns

- understand that flexible people are not necessarily healthier than inflexible people

- realize how many people are out of touch with their bodies

- maximize the intelligence of tissue, plasticity of tissue, and capacity for change

- know that body and mind have the intelligence to heal and thrive

- understand the differences, sometimes radical, between one side of the body and the other

- appreciate the broad ranges in tissue texture. No two bodies exhibit the same texture (this can be said of minds)

- know that moving a limb can be a gross or delicately refined action

- work with involuntary rhythms

- have an opportunity to recognize the benefits of an understated approach

- are aware of a bigger picture.

Yoga teachers appear to make more of an investment in consciousness and its quality, although this may be a generalization. Osteopathic schools do not cover the great sages of the East. But osteopathy's founder, Andrew Taylor Still, was not only an inspired doctor but also a spiritually oriented healer. "*I quote no authors but God and experience*" (Still 1892/1986). It is a personal choice. Some osteopathic healers, due to the direction of their practice, are attracted to the nature and quality of consciousness and a more universal perspective. It comes up, and they feel it. Insight and realization can thrive within the one-to-one healing space. There are yoga teachers who could learn from osteopathic sensitivity and osteopaths who could learn from yoga's insight and realization.

The disc

The consequences were inevitable. My back pain returned with a vengeance. Persistent overstretching had at first resolved intermittent pain but had aggravated an L4/L5 disc. As the muscles tightened to protect the area I would stretch for initial relief, but put additional strain on the ligaments and posterior disc. Personal experience taught me about extreme unremitting lumbar and sciatic pain and muscular hypotrophy. Turning over in bed at night, on pain killers, could take 10 minutes. People were calling me for treatment and I could hardly walk to the door to let them in. When I did work, I had to support my weight on the treatment table while treating others for far less serious conditions. I sought help from one of my osteopathic teachers who was an authority on the minutiae of spinal mechanics. He misdiagnosed, called in an assistant, and between them they performed a "two-man technique" – one pulls a leg and the other whacks the pelvis with a mighty clunk. I was traumatized but still in one piece. Another lesson. A disc problem cannot be effectively directly treated. I rested. When clients presented with disc issues I had an understanding, empathy, and confidence, which I would not have had were it not for my own experience.

A woman's touch

Following several weeks of rest, improved but still in pain, I saw a cranial practitioner. She was more than effective. Twenty minutes with her hand under my sacrum got me on the road to recovery. Things improved from that moment. I felt ready to get back to yoga, but it would need a different approach.

I went to see my Russian friend Mina Semyon, a yoga teacher who had been a key figure in the group around R. D. Laing. She had a considered approach, working quietly and gently in each position. I went for some helpful sessions. Mina, on her recent 80th birthday, sat in the middle of the floor in full lotus playing the guitar and singing Russian songs. She has published two books: *The Distracted Centipede: A Yoga Experience* and *Yoga Stories for Healthy Living*. She continues to teach and entertain people with her humor, stories, songs, and insight.

PROLOGUE *continued*

Sandra Sabatini, Lolly, and I approached Vanda Scaravelli's house overlooking Florence. We had a life-size model of a spine and pelvis. Vanda was delighted with the gift, continually pointing to the tailbone. "You see, you see! Its length. Its location. Don't forget the tail." We had met Sandra in London through Mary Stewart, a dynamic and transformative Iyengar teacher. We began to work with Sandra, a long-term student of Vanda's, and enjoyed several of her retreats in Italy. Sandra is a charismatic and generous teacher who focuses on the breath. We combined our understanding and ran a few workshops together. Vanda was interested in my osteopathic understanding of her work. When I was in Italy teaching with Sandra, she would take me to see Vanda.

Vanda Scaravelli had a radically different approach to the body involving gravity and breath. She had been a student of Iyengar and had learnt about the breath from Desikachar. The story goes she had adapted the work when teaching "the exercises" to Krishnamurti. Vanda's approach was appealing and effective. I made special trips see her, about six times over two years, each time for about four or five days. I learnt a lot from her. I will always be grateful for Vanda's generosity on all levels. Her book *Awakening the Spine* reflects her work. I had her message, and now was being drawn in another direction.

And then

Consciousness beckoned. My body continued to change, and mind and consciousness followed. I wanted to talk about it, share it, and found myself referring more and more to *how we are,* our internal behavior, and conditioning. I began highlighting yoga's vastness, its scope, and intimate connection to all that we are and do. It was not planned. It just kept coming up in classes and workshops. I began to synthesize the physical focus with my experience of the depth, range, and power of undisturbed consciousness. Going deeply into sensation and the mind had a transformative effect on all aspects of experience.

As yoga teachers, what qualifications do we need to approach issues such as relationship, behavior, and insight? Psychology, the ancient texts, sutras, and what others have said are enlightening and useful. We appreciate the insight and wisdom of others and may refer to inspiring minds, but their purpose is to stir something in us, something that is already there. First-hand, subjective experience of ourselves, and ourselves in relationship to others, is a fundamental key to understanding. We understand the nature of relationship by relating in the moment, by being attentive to mental and emotional nuances, and *sensing* shifts at the time. The nature of relationship is in front of us. It is something that is happening that is alive. We work with it in ourselves and with others on a daily basis.

Joy comes with the realization that we inherently *know*, that everyone inherently *knows*. Our students *know* and at times may *know* more clearly than we do. It is a shared experience. Clarity surfaces when we navigate distractions. We are not telling people how to be, simply highlighting the impediments and, if the interest is there, the potential for change along the way.

Now

I ceased practicing as an osteopath 20 years ago. We moved out of London and took a year out to renovate a house in Sussex. Soon after, I returned to my work as a yoga teacher. The depth and scope of teaching appears endless. Understanding and sensitivity continue to grow and insight flourishes. In years past, some viewed yoga teaching as "not a proper job." Nowadays teaching yoga can be a mainstream profession, if that is what we want it to be. It is competitive and there are many variations. But, yes, there is one yoga and, yes, it resides in each of us. We can allow ourselves distractions, but ultimately we return to our own experience and the inspiration it gives us to teach.

The meaning of yoga has never been clearer. Uncertainties hover, fade, surface, and fade again, but much less so, and my relationship to them has changed. I respect them as an essential aspect of change. I have learnt so much from students, from being with others who have taught me kindness and patience. Without these qualities, things will not work out because the tension that ignores or supresses them pervades one's entire experience. I no longer look for explanations as to why some things happen in classes as they do or seek new students, although they come. *The Original Body* was published in 2015. This book is where I am now. The healing continues.

Lolly and I have been together for 47 years. In one way we feel we are just beginning. Her work continues to thrive: educating pregnant women and their partners and teaching yoga teachers how to work with pregnancy and birth. The pleasant anticipation of seeing familiar and unfamiliar faces in a group never leaves me. The wisdom, insight and love that bonds us with our students, with one another and beyond, cannot be captured or planned. I'm about to begin a workshop. The best is yet to come!

Introduction

This book suggests that sensory experience is the key to profound insight. It invites teachers to share with their students the clarity, mental space, and basic wisdom that emerge from an awakening body. Experience shows that enhancing and transcending physical sensation brings lucid insight. Physical approaches create change but a potential exists for an infinitely deep mind–body relationship. Physical practice influences the mind *and* invites consciousness to act as a sensory tool, leading to profound transformation.

Yoga's bodywork is powerfully effective. Its approach to personal conditioning and its bearing on the bigger picture has a potency rarely found elsewhere. This may be because Eastern culture is one of extremes. The Eastern approach to personal transformation is exhaustive in its attempt to penetrate conditioned minds, and may demand a discipline unpalatable for Western appetites. In comparison, Western approaches appear to float above the possibilities that lie beneath the surface. Modern yoga may draw criticism for being shallow because the deeper tensions surrounding our conditioning may appear impenetrable. Perhaps deeper change involves too much work or is considered unnecessary.

Practicing alone is in line with tradition and an essential aspect of a teacher's work. We also encourage students to develop a personal practice and many do. But the creative communion of group work can be just as, if not more, transformative. Being *in it* with the group maximizes our presence, our guidance, and the impact of our voice. The "What Lies Beneath" courses for teachers have been particularly effective for reaching inward as participants discover previously inaccessible aspects of themselves. The courses have shown the value of sustained attention to the surface tissues and demonstrated a parallel effect on the psychological and emotional areas of our work.

Deeper transformation arises as a consequence of a profound communication between teacher and students. The most frequent remarks from teachers attending courses are: "I have not felt that before," "the level of connectivity was surprising," "my internal behavior is changing," and "I now understand the potential depth of yoga." The feedback suggests that a heightened understanding can be used for teaching *at the time of its emergence*. Experiential teaching and learning is based on what is *there*, how we *are*, and what we *notice*, moment by moment.

Classical yoga introduced a quality of mind associated with a deep, broad, and lucid consciousness. It would be honoring yoga and ourselves to approach body-oriented practice with a depth that might stand up to the scrutiny of traditional practice. Approaching the body with depth *in mind* draws focused attention to our inner life. What is depth and how does it feel? Physical depth is felt within the finer sensations of tissue, but the total yoga experience invites an immeasurable depth of consciousness.

No one, even today, knows what consciousness actually is, understands how it comes about, or how it is experienced. No one really knows what experience is or how we experience anything. The neurochemical basis for experience may be known, but science has yet to understand the connection between the neurochemistry and the experience itself. The gap in understanding provides the space for speculation and the possibility of an ever-deepening creativity.

As practice deepens, we pass through the density of conditioned experience into *less-ness*, the unified *one with everything* experience. Experience beyond unification is not easily described and loses its power in the description, hence the mystic's investment in the unknown. The yoga experience, if anything, *is* the experience of the unknown, if the unknown can be an experience. The quandary is that as something is experienced it becomes known, a phenomenon the physicist David Bohm and others describe as the nonmanifest becoming manifest. While science invests in the "yet to be known" in a quest to understand it, yoga's pursuit of an unconditioned mind thrives on the unknown, and is a pursuit that promises infinite possibilities.

Shifts in consciousness, the fertility of creative insight, and the transformative power of unification are a consequence of releasing the grip of the ego and dissolving habitual conditioning. Awakening to the deeper self is the first stage toward experiencing a bigger picture as opposed to the *idea* of it. While researchers on the possibility of universal intelligence maintain by their own admission that their theories are based on assumptions, the subjective process of going inward stimulates a "universal experience." This is a common occurrence in group work as the group field takes effect. As we refine sensation, we are drawn into a profound understanding that can be shared with those we teach.

This book suggests that inherent insight is a powerful teaching tool that is released by combining physical sensation with focused attention on consciousness. Teachers can invite their students to listen to their own experience more closely as the tissues reveal the relationship between an awakening body and a dynamic quality of consciousness. Students begin to reveal their own insights as emergent wisdom inspires debate. We can always draw more attention to attention itself and to the inherent qualities of insight. Yoga is the science of the individual engaged in personal inquiry, a project that can be enhanced by group participation. Mutuality is work in progress, is not finite, and is beyond structures. There is no point at which we can say *that's it* because *that's it* is caught in the past, without movement or possibility.

We can teach yoga as bodywork and deepen the physical approach, or we can teach the essence of yoga *via* the body and deepen consciousness. We can research the nature of consciousness by acknowledging the body as its material base and the sensory route for realizing alternative states of mind. We can appreciate sensation as a profound and abiding meditation.

While researching for this book, I discovered that some of the basic concepts put forward by modern physics were known to me through my own practice. Personal insights also resonated with those recorded through the centuries (but not because of them). Most of the text in this book springs from my own insight. We should trust and express our insights.

Some external information is relevant to personal inquiry and may include physiology, psychology, quantum theory, spirituality, or anything concerning personal transformation. I have kept references to a minimum because much of the available information is either superfluous or too complex to support progress. I have repeatedly acknowledged a few past and present authorities whom I respect, and who confess they *don't know*, yet sustain

INTRODUCTION *continued*

the inspiration to *find out*. I have no scientific evidence to support the reality that going 'more' deeply into oneself has the transformative and powerful effect that it does. Personal experience suggests that more depth implies more transformation. The testimony of my own experience and of those who work with me has been sufficient. If yoga is to cultivate a deeply relaxed and lucid mind, it requires an intensity of focus needed to negotiate directly with the patterns associated with our conditioning. This intensity can be highlighted by the group field.

Addressing physical sensation and dissolving conditioned patterns refines consciousness. While the spine is recognized for its depth and its role in transformation, a transcendent consciousness can be realized through the tissues due to their continuity, accessibility, sensory presence, and their role in the formation of the ego. This book highlights the surface of the body as a door to profound realization and suggests that heightened sensation transforms consciousness.

Deeper Still is not an instruction manual but points to the potential depth and impact of what we do. Its observations, suggestions and insights consider the profound aspects of the yoga experience. Yoga may mean different things to different people. In essence, yoga is a living experience. Ideally the means to realizing this experience should be as direct and simple as possible and requires listening to one's own experience as it arises.

Through authentic embodiment modern yoga can find its way to an experience known to practitioners through the ages. But guiding others is based on an unknown element upon which all creativity is founded. We are the authority and, having reached the limitations of what others have said, can propel ourselves into the creative field of space, consciousness, and insight.

For centuries yoga has pointed to our innermost place as having no content. Its teachers have described the experience in terms best suited to their environment and culture. Regardless of culture, we can all realize this space and the benefits of doing so. We can write our own story, develop our own script, and take others with us. More depth, more space, and more unknowns await us. Use this book to confirm what you inherently know. We have a deep, abiding relationship with the creative unknown. Inherent insight can be shared as it emerges. We are students of our own nature.

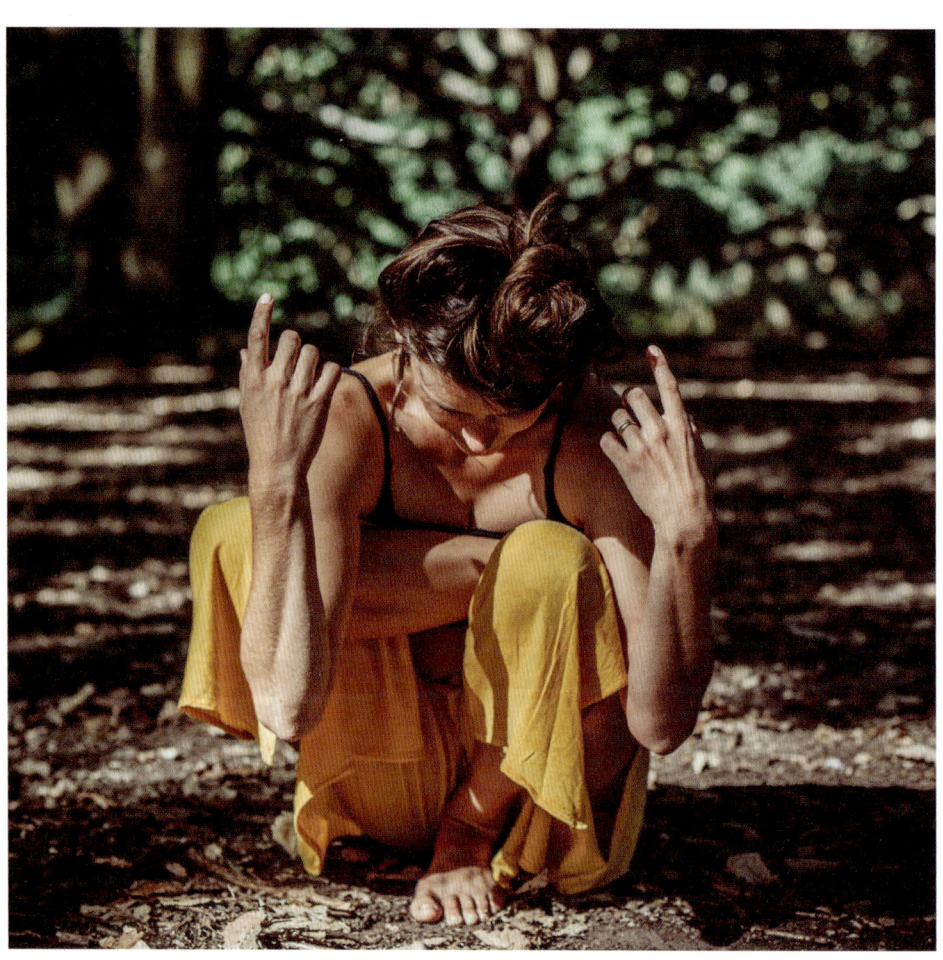

THE REALITY

The reality of yoga is unseen and beyond shapes or extensions. The reality concerns an awareness of all that we are and might be. We are the reality.

The reality of yoga proposes that we are asleep and yet to awaken to an abiding sense of totality. Initially developed to transcend our conditioning, yoga demanded an austere approach. The exercises are effective but the problem of conditioned minds is deeply embedded. For some, the reality may be the pleasure of the bodywork, for others it may be a deepening sense of self, or a shift in habitual behavior. The philosophy not the bodywork has sustained yoga's appeal over many centuries. At its core, yoga's reality confronts and transcends our limits. We are aware of the physical limitations but generally unaware of the limitations of a conditioned consciousness. Addressing the *problem of us* takes more than bodywork, but our attraction to the sensory aspect can be used as a door to a deeper and sustainable transformation on other levels.

The classical yoga practitioners were primarily concerned with the quality of consciousness. An inner inquiry has encouraged individuals to engage in intense personal experimentation for thousands of years. We may be as much in need of this now as at any other time in our history. We may have tasted yoga's depth, had light bulb moments, but a more sustainable change is possible. Can we provide an undiluted transformative practice? It is not surprising the West has embraced the physical aspect, as the Eastern approach is elusive and demanding. Much of the philosophy taken at face value is unrealistic.

We may not aspire to enlightenment, but class work experiences show that a deeper transformation is not far away from everyday consciousness. We can work with the body while giving the mind the attention it deserves and work with the mind while giving the body the same courtesy. We might acknowledge the Dalai Lama's observation that unhappiness abounds in societies that appear to have most things at their fingertips and follow his suggestion that we might give more attention to our inner life. We can take the mind's turbulence and the grip of the ego more seriously while attending to the body.

Distinctions between traditional and modern yoga do not change the fact that we can take the mind deeply into the body. Sensation opens other possibilities. The body as

Chapter 1

the way in distinguishes a bodywork class from something more profound. Yoga as the science of *being* helps us function from the present with a vested interest in the quality of our consciousness and internal behavior.

Yoga gives us the tools and the terminology to describe its scope and depth but its potential can be limited by its methodology and knowledge. We can call on anatomy, philosophy, or Sanskrit at any time, but in the thick of practice knowledge falls by the wayside and information inhibits transcendent moments. Avoiding the weight of knowledge involves dropping knowledge as it comes up. Space should remain open for inspired and creative insight to emerge. Information plays its role but also blocks the potential for lucid observations.

What if?

What if we had no choice but to follow our own experience? What if we had not heard of Iyengar, Freud, Jung, or Krishnamurti? What if there were no life sciences, philosophy, Eastern or Greek thought? What if we had not discovered the wisdom of Patanjali, Buddha, Rajneesh, and others? What if there were no books, courses, methods, or teachers? What if, in the first instance, we could only rely on personal investigation and *then* look at what others have said? What if we were our own starting point minus the expectations accompanying external knowledge? What if we only had our feeling, thinking mind and body as we perceive it? What if *we* were our only resource?

Would we discover our conditioning or dullness, awaken sensation, lucidity and consciousness, realize the value of confronting resistance and discover a new depth of understanding? Would we benefit from a personal practice undisturbed by theory, anatomical detail, or past ideas? Initial guidance is essential. We have all been guided, and we guide others, but the deeper we go the more obvious it becomes that the essence is realized by personal discovery.

Conditioning

We are all conditioned by our past. Conditioning is the camouflage that disguises our potential. It can be productive to discuss conditioning with groups. Conditioning expresses itself in many ways but is generally reflected by an unsettled mind and a need for identification and attachment. Some traits are inherited, but our environment plays its part in determining how and to what intensity we are conditioned. Conditioning is defined as *a learned behavior built up into a set of responses that have become part of our general conduct* (internal and external). Conditioning is influenced by culture, belief systems, family, education, and exposure to the influence of others over an extended period, particularly around the perinatal period and when young.

The fact of being conditioned is nothing new, but it is a matter of degree. At worst conditioning may instill irrational fear, lack of confidence, low self-esteem, or compulsive behavior. On other levels conditioning may inhibit personal freedom, ease, spontaneity, a sense of unification with others, and the ability to realize creative authenticity and insight, or an ability to experience the fullness of life.

Positive conditioning, such as socialization, is necessary and teaches us how to coexist with and relate to others. Negative conditioning

The Reality

creates fixed patterns that may go unnoticed and impede personal potential. We have learnt to inhibit reactive feelings and emotion. If instilled early enough, inhibitions sink beneath awareness. Observing our internal behavior highlights the fact of our conditioning.

Over many centuries, practitioners have sought to address conditioned ways of being. Turbulent minds, the incessancy of thought, and untoward internal behavior have been the focus of attention throughout the ages. We may condition each thought and feeling because they are filtered through a screen of conditioning, hence yoga's focus on addressing the incessancy of thought and reinstating a calm and spatial mind. *Conditioning is the calcification of the soul.*

Practice acts as a lens, magnifying internal behavior and slowing us down, so that we may "catch" the mind as it veers and jerks from one thing to the next. This is made possible by practices intended to transform our way of being, as opposed to those with fitness as a primary aim. The first step is to wake up to the fact of being conditioned. However useful we are as teachers, we should acknowledge conditioning in ourselves and in those who come to us. We are all conditioned in one way or another, some of us more than others, and through no fault of our own. Some suggest that the consciousness of all mankind is negatively conditioned. Yoga practitioners, including teachers, may be conditioned by yoga. We may have a subconscious resistance to moving on from a specific mold or sustain an attachment to a practice that has lost its effectiveness. We may be caught in a method for security, convenience, marketing, or the feeling that it is what students want.

The need to address conditioning is accepted in the West as a factor in our quest for well-being. What may be less accepted is the *extent* of the grip that conditioning has on our minds and internal behavior. Enlightened individuals are aware of their conditioned responses as they engage with life and with themselves. They see things coming and have the timing to field certain aspects of their behavior. This understanding is a feature and a consequence of meditation.

Even when we recognize it in ourselves, we cannot always address conditioning directly. Due to its hold, conditioned patterning requires practices deep enough to release it. The conditioned mind cannot decondition itself by itself. Highlighting and transforming our inner state requires profound, focused attention and the appropriate bodywork.

We can address conditioning and open a door to something deeper. We can address *the problem of us* in line with traditional practice, by working in simple postures with a sensitivity that disperses habitual patterns. Basic positions have the additional advantage that students can stay in them for extended periods. Self-observation is made easy when we are not distracted by perfecting positions, but can use them as meditations.

We can inject physical work with a deeply focused and sustainably attentive mind. Light bulb moments are transient stages of deconditioning, temporary enlightening experiences during an ongoing process of change, confirming we are headed in the right direction.

Chapter 1

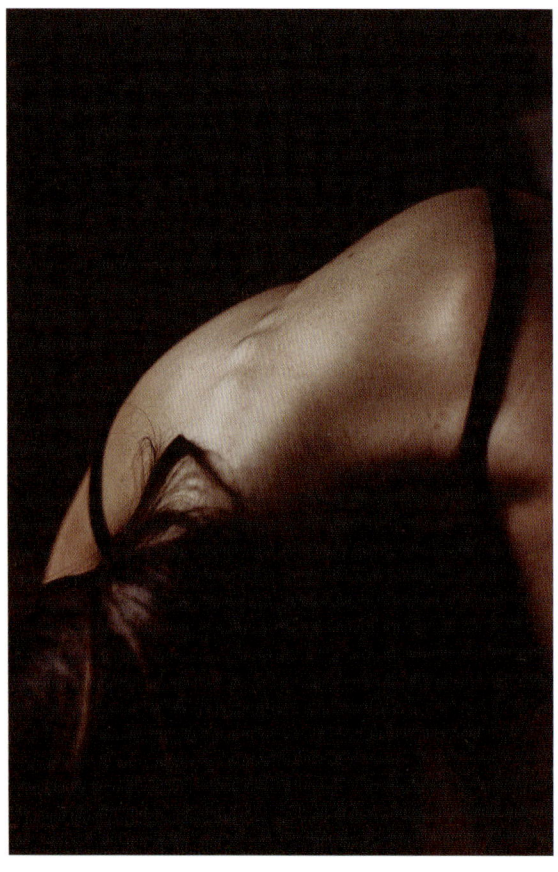

Highlighting and transforming our inner state requires profound, focused attention and the appropriate bodywork.

Awakening

There are some who are awake even while asleep, and then there are those who, apparently awake, are deeply asleep.
(Lalla in Feuerstein 1997)

Sleepiness refers to impeded clarity, dullness, lack of awareness, and habitual mental heaviness. A subtle *closing down* of consciousness may indicate a cutoff against unwanted feelings, a defensive response to one's environment, lack of stimulation, ongoing stress, or a mind that just cannot let go of itself. Awakening has been the aim of spiritual practice throughout the ages. We are asleep and have yet to realize our true awakened nature. Awakening may appear unnecessary *until we feel awakened*. In retrospect we realize we have been enclosed in a shroud of limited awareness. Awakening the deeper fusion between body and mind awakens other areas. As the divide heals and we *break out*, we awaken attention, awareness, sensory appreciation, spatial sensation, and emotional sensitivity. We awaken lucidity, presence, consciousness, and an understanding of the profound nature of relationship.

The degree of awakening depends on the approach and how people receive it. It takes time to revitalize the sensory system. Understanding the nature of living tissue is relevant when we *feel it*. The fact that awakening tissue affects consciousness is due to the enhanced function of nerves and biochemistry, but the experience is beyond neurological or chemical understanding. We *feel* lucid because the sensory system wakes up. The quality of wakefulness is enhanced by being attentive to sensation, not by imagining the details of sensory conveyance. The sensory system is a continuum, skin to spinal cord, synapse to synapse, fluid to nerve, and tissue to tissue, but we work with feeling itself and are more sensitive when free from the clutter of physiological information and when we give ourselves to sensation.

The Reality

As tissues awaken, we awaken personal attributes, creativity, and anything that could be described as a spiritual dimension. We awaken our experience.

Well-trodden paths

Habitual practice follows well-trodden paths that inhibit new discoveries. Habit restrains deeper exploration. At any given moment we can choose between covering the same ground in the same way or consciously entering deeper levels of experience. Choosing emptiness over thought, presence over anticipation, or calmness over flux is a practice. Following well-trodden paths is inevitable, but we can use familiar postures for going ever more deeply. Positions follow accustomed pathways, but we can use them to enter tissue more deeply and sink beneath familiar layers. How we respond to deeper inquiry holds the key to understanding, and bypasses recourse to any authority other than oneself. We tend to favor familiar paths because they work, but conditioning can draw us into habitual patterns. Conditioned patterns affect how we move, think, and behave and instil a resistance to change. We dissolve patterns by addressing resistance.

Resistance

There is a fine line between tissue resistance and tissue engagement. Regardless of range of movement, resistance in the body softens, opens, and spreads at the touch of the mind. It may take time for students to understand this quality and its effect on consciousness.

Resistance supports habitual patterns and features in all body–mind work and provides the focus for transcending limitations. The word *resist* means to *withstand* and *the opposition offered by one body to the pressure or movement of another*. Withstanding or resisting unwanted feelings or emotions employs physical pressure to inhibit the feeling. We have *become* resistant to sensations associated with unwanted experiences. Resistance is a central factor in psychoanalysis, psychotherapy, and bioenergetics. A period of resistance precedes the release of repressed feelings connected to past experiences. Emotional resistance runs parallel to the memories stored in the body and inhibits tissue motility and spontaneity. Resistance has many textures and nuances and differs widely between individuals. Resistance may pervade the tissues anywhere or everywhere. Addressing resistance involves engaging with it.

Teachers are well placed to understand resistance. We feel it in our bodies and notice it in our minds. A particular sensitivity is needed to discover and dissolve deeper resistances. Hidden resistance may involve past trauma, postural factors, habit, conditioning, or anxiety. Approaching resistance should acknowledge that consciousness opens with the body. Consciousness recognizes physical resistance as a part of itself. Patterns grip deeply and removing them requires an equally deep approach. Resistance is creative when we seek it out, engage it, and pass through it.

Addressing resistance is a transformative experience. Tissue changes texture, the mind clears, consciousness becomes more lucid,

Chapter 1

and conditioning dissolves. Doubt, anticipation, and anxiety disperse as we tune to the nuances of ever-changing tension. Creative engagement leads us away from our familiar selves into a deeper reality. The greater the depth, the further away we find ourselves. As an ongoing process, transformation moves from one state into the next. As each state consolidates, a door to the next state opens. Gentle, considered, sensitive, and responsive engagement reveals another reality.

Anxiety matters

Awakening sensation can arouse anxiety as habitual patterns surface. Anxiety is an insidious feature of conditioning. There is a fine line between anxiety and fear. Anxiety is connected to a vague sense of apprehension, while fear is usually an emotional response to a known threat. We may be afraid *of* something or anxious *about* something. Although fear may relate to a known threat, psychological fear, as a condition in itself, can pervade our experience and seem out of proportion to its cause. Anxiety and fear are appropriate when proportional to circumstances that provoke them. The crossover between fear and anxiety may not always be clear, but both are felt in the body. The intensity of the sensations depends upon circumstances and personal conditioning. Fear takes many forms and is not always obvious. We might be unaware of a subtle unease within the background of awareness *until we notice it*. We may be fearful of fear itself. Irrational anxiety is the feeling of being threatened by an unknown source.

We should be interested in anxiety, acknowledging it in ourselves and in those we teach. Groups agree that anxiety matters and are willing to discuss it. Anxiety can surface as we work through resistance and transcend conditioned patterns. Freud suggested that a primary anxiety is a consequence of the trauma of birth (not birth trauma but the actual trauma of being born) followed by an anxiety about separation from the mother. He also suggested that fear of death was a root cause of all fear. Like Freud, Wilhelm Reich and his student Alexander Lowen, the pioneers of bioenergetics, proposed that a deep anxiety arose from the suppression of physical desires and needs coming from the unconscious and rooted in the body. Krishnamurti suggested that (irrational) fear and anxiety arose from thought, proposing that thought, when in (or out of) control, leads to an anxiety about something. We can pin fear and anxiety on anything. Fear of relationships, fear of loss, fear of pain, fear of things that might never happen. Anxiety may be handed down through generations. Genetic anxiety is common in cultures that inherit the memory of the misfortunes of their people. Anxiety is pathological when out of proportion to the situation that created it.

How is your relationship with anxiety? How does it feel in your body? How irrational, pervasive, or well founded is anxiety? Does it arise for no apparent reason? Are you aware of its subtlety? Fear and anxiety invade the tissues, the breath, and the gut, and range from mild to overwhelming sensations. Where does anxiety come from, how much has it been instilled by conditioning, how does it influence our behavior, and how do we deal with it? Anxiety may come unexpectedly and vary in intensity. We can read about anxiety, understand its biochemistry,

The Reality

listen to others about their anxiety, or understand it through direct experience.

On one level or another no one is exempt. With this in mind, plus the potential tension arising from postural work, we have our work cut out. Addressing resistance while sustaining the sensitivity needed to pick up and dissolve yet to be discovered patterns is the ultimate exercise.

The Swiss cultural philosopher Jean Gebser had an interesting view on anxiety. In his extraordinary book, *The Ever-Present Origin*, he wrote:

Trust is the positive form of anxiety while hope is the positive form of fear … fear and hope are phenomena of insecurity which the mind relates to the future … But anxiety and trust are inceptual phenomena, latent in themselves and in us when we are conscious of them; at least in the Christian view, anxiety can turn to trust and consequently innermost security. (Gebser 1949/1985)

Converting anxiety into trust is the essential factor in establishing an atmosphere most suited for transcendence. An underlying anxiety runs through the fabric of society. We have learnt not to trust, which is a counterproductive attitude in body–mind work. As students arrive, we can acknowledge trust as the essential ingredient promoting positive qualities and dispelling underlying anxiety. Some teachers may be more anxious than some of their students. Anxiety around teaching is commonplace. New and established teachers can be anxious about unfamiliar groups, stiffening up (losing it), exposure, standing before others, or coming up with the goods, which may evoke a lifelong anxiety instilled by factors beyond our control. We can insulate ourselves with the security of a familiar method, but the best teaching is beyond methods, inspires students, and teaches us more about ourselves.

Imposing resistance on the body can stir up anxiety or even fear. Some students panic as they engage the hamstrings. Negotiating tissue resistance is the essential consideration and is difficult to teach. Negotiation is different for each person because texture is so personal, but the feelings that arise are similar. Tension can be fear, and fear is tension, hence the need to go slowly and find ways of dissolving resistance that do not create but dispel anxiety, if and when it presents itself.

Iyengar found it difficult to teach the degree of surrender he expected from his students. He discovered that Westerners did not have the required mental or physical compliance. How do we transcend resistance? It is not an all-or-nothing issue but concerns finding *that place*! The key is in *lightly engaging and being with* the tissue and proceeding from there.

Adjusting consciousness and tissue engagement to each other is an art. Some feelings are so commonplace they may not be associated with anxiety, but if turbulence arises you may notice elements of background anxiety. Practice does not completely evaporate anxiety in the longer term. Anxiety can return with seemingly more intensity because of the marked contrast between transcendent relaxation and unexpected fearfulness. We can take the edge off. A more sustainable outcome requires a deeply measured and patient focus.

Chapter 1

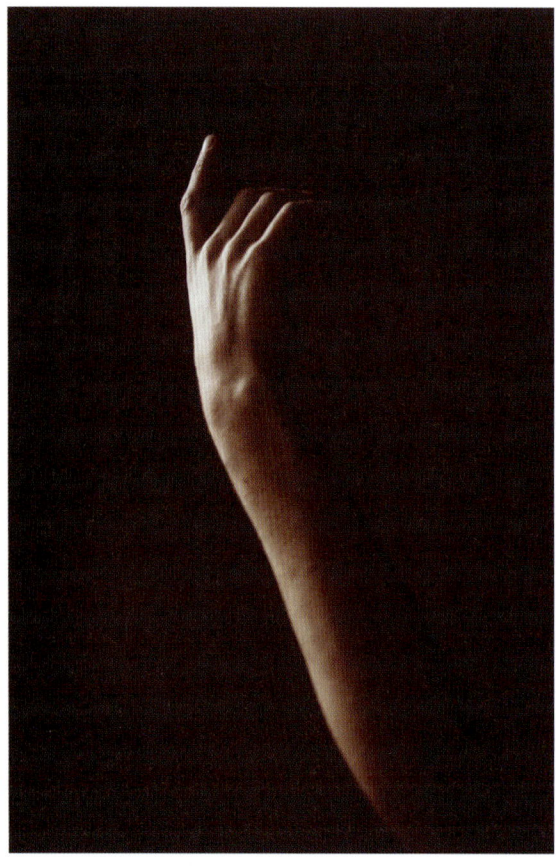

A place within lies quietly beneath everything we perceive as physical, emotional, or psychological.

Freedom and anxiety

In drawing our attention to background anxiety, practice also frees us from it. However, there is an anxiety concerning freedom itself. Some students experience anxiety stemming from *a loss of self*. Transcending resistance and dissolving habitual patterns may set us adrift in a sea of emptiness.

The Danish philosopher Søren Kierkegaard referred to this kind of experience in his book *The Concept of Anxiety*, suggesting that we court freedom but reject the uncertainty and insecurity that come with it. We reject the infinite and settle for the stability of the finite. We inhibit the possibilities because opening ourselves to the freedom of the unknown creates anxiety. Kierkegaard suggested that an ambiguity between existential anxiety and freedom is a precondition of life. He wrote: "Learning to know anxiety is an adventure which every man has to affront. He therefore who has learned rightly to be in anxiety has learned the most important thing" (Kierkegaard 1844/1980).

Kierkegaard's understanding points to the *void* of practice. An unaccustomed freedom from oneself invites the anxiety of detachment. This can be palpable in groups that are moving through a transitional experience. As we slip out of familiar patterns an anxiety may arise around a newfound freedom based on less self and less identity. Learning to hold the balance provides an enlightening experience. Creativity involves stepping into the unknown and accepting the sense of unconditioned liberation. Passing through resistance, observing it spread and soften, dissolves associated anxiety. Teaching this to others demands constant reference and patience. The following quote by Jean Gebser describes a positive side to anxiety and gives an indication of where we might find ourselves.

Anxiety inevitably comes about where the lack of an alternative becomes consciously or unconsciously evident in a particular attitude or stance where it reflects the

THE REALITY

impotence rather than the potency of the particular attitude ... anxiety is always the first sign that a mutation is coming to the end of its expressive and effective possibilities causing new powers to accumulate which, because they are thwarted, create a narrows [sic] or constriction. At the culmination point of anxiety these powers liberate themselves, and this liberation is always synonymous with a new mutation. In this sense anxiety, [sic] is the great birth giver. (Gebser 1949/1985)

Discomfort

Resistance in the tissues is ideally soft, pliant, and responsive and can be dispersed by the slightest suggestion from the mind. It takes time to reveal this quality which is dependent on the quality of consciousness. If discomfort gets in the way, to what extent should we back off? Students find the balance elusive. Should we work with discomfort or avoid it entirely? Discomfort can create anxiety and anxiety feeds discomfort. There is a difference between creating discomfort through force or effort and revealing *hidden discomfort* relating to patterns of conditioned tension. We must be careful. We cannot ask others to work through discomfort. Forty years ago, during the "strong stretching days," a friend pointed out that the Mongol warriors, the night before battle, would work on their bodies with a small tool designed to eradicate the pain they associated with fear. Considering their reputation and success, the process was obviously successful. Nevertheless, pain and discomfort should be respected and avoided.

Painful experiences are woven into the tissues. Memories of past physical and emotional trauma often surface as tension dissolves. Sensation is entirely subjective. For some people stiffness feels like pain, and for others pain feels like stiffness. Exchanging sensation with someone might show their pain as mild discomfort. Conversely, someone else's ache may feel like pain. It is a matter of degree. Stronger sensation can bring out an inherent anxiety in the tissues or create an anxiety proportional to the intensity of the resistance.

Gentle engagement provides a door to space and realization. Sensations of resistance become pleasurable. Following through on discomfort requires experience and sensitivity, involving a moment-to-moment refinement. If tissue remains unyielding, the reminder to back off cannot be overemphasized. Alexander Lowen put it like this: "If tension develops in situations in which the anticipation of pleasurable release is not possible, anxiety is experienced" (Lowen 1958). His statement implies an edge that promises transcendent release, something the tissues understand more than we do.

Dealing with occasional discomfort related to resistance can only be understood personally. How we go about it is a priority in group work. Passing through our own restrictions clears the way for advising others. We can guide others toward their potential by helping them to find and sustain the fine balance between the discovery of tension and its release. If you go to a bodyworker who locates a sensitive area you might suggest he ease off but also ask him to continue if you know the effect will be positive.

Chapter 1

Living tissue acquires habitual tension and a residue of associated toxins. More sensitive areas indicate fascial gumming, adhesions, and contractive soft tissue. When opened, these areas release energy into the entire body, into the mind, and into consciousness. It is essential to discuss the pros and cons of resistance with groups, as they learn how to use their mental focus to pass through tension and discover what lies on the other side. Practice is most effective when we dissolve and pass through something. The key issue is what to dissolve and how to pass through it. We can introduce a physical approach that awakens and disperses conditioned patterns.

A teacher's reality

What do we see before us? A collection of fascial organizations, people performing exercises, or thinking, feeling individuals with an inherent potential for discovery, innovation, and transformation? Based on our experience, we introduce others to a deeper sensitivity and work with their sensations, emotions, individuality, impediments, anxieties, and expectations. Assumptions are counterproductive. An awareness that everyone may not be having the same experience at the same time provides an atmosphere of possibility for the whole group. We may have the anatomy and the philosophy but need the mental space. The reality of teaching involves recognizing our own conditioning in relation to that of others, which is an essential acknowledgment for showing others how to address their conscious or unconscious resistances.

We observe a group's tension, sense it in our bodies, assess resistance, effort, calmness, and weakness, and may move amongst students, making suggestions here or there. We can also *be in it with them*. The group field takes on a powerful feel when we join them and lead from there. We can go directly to the mind as we enter the tissue. We can pass through all the feelings, thoughts, and activity that produce selves. Whatever the mental content, whatever is *there*, we can penetrate and dissolve the mind's content and the physical tension with focused attention. We can apply this anywhere at any time.

Going into one's self involves passing through the tension of one's self. Traditional yoga sees reality as realization, the manifestation of insightful reality, an unconditioned experience. Perceptions are free from the veil of "I am" as we get out of our own way. When we get caught up, deeper practice mitigates emotional reactions to old patterns.

Deeper practice

Practice tempers conditioning and deeper practice has the most impact. Conditioning is addressed by being attentive, by unobsessively noticing how we are. Deeper physical work is direct and immediate and sustains the action that brings us face-to-face with ourselves. Sensation and consciousness hold the interest and quieten fluctuating minds. Addressing physical patterns coexistent with conditioning necessitates engaging the tension that perpetuates our idea of ourselves.

The Reality

The essential aspects of what we do lack material substance. We cannot see or hold the faculty of attention but feel its expression. Consciousness is supported by neurological and biochemical activity but we cannot see consciousness itself. We can only see its result. We cannot see so-called enlightenment, nor identify what awareness actually is. We can identify expressions of behavior but cannot see behavior itself. Thought, experience, and feeling are nonmaterial qualities without material substance. Personal qualities have no substance but we see their expression in behavior. Although you and I are materially *being*, we cannot see *being*, in spite of the fact that we obviously *are*. Yoga cannot be seen but is experienced as a quality.

Discovering deeper roots involves nonmaterial phenomena such as awareness, attention, and consciousness. We work through the material substance of the body to enhance our nonmaterial qualities. The fact that qualities of being are without material substance enables us to operate from a place of emptiness. There is no conflict at the deeper level. In the process of *what happens*, everything passing through the mind is a sequence of witnessed events moving through an expansive consciousness.

We cannot imitate authenticity, or realization. We cannot teach sensation directly but can describe it and invite others to seek it out. The deeper we go, the more possibilities reveal themselves. *The problem of us* is addressed *by* us: a starting point never reaching a conclusion. Ongoing awareness and attention take our discoveries into the field of teaching.

A place inside us lies quietly beneath everything we perceive as physical, emotional, or psychological. We may not sustain it for long periods but can hover gently at its edge, peer into it, and observe its vastness. An interpretation of reality acknowledges all experience as grounded in a physical sense of self. Minds and bodies change each other as sensation gains entry into the reality of an expansive subjectivity.

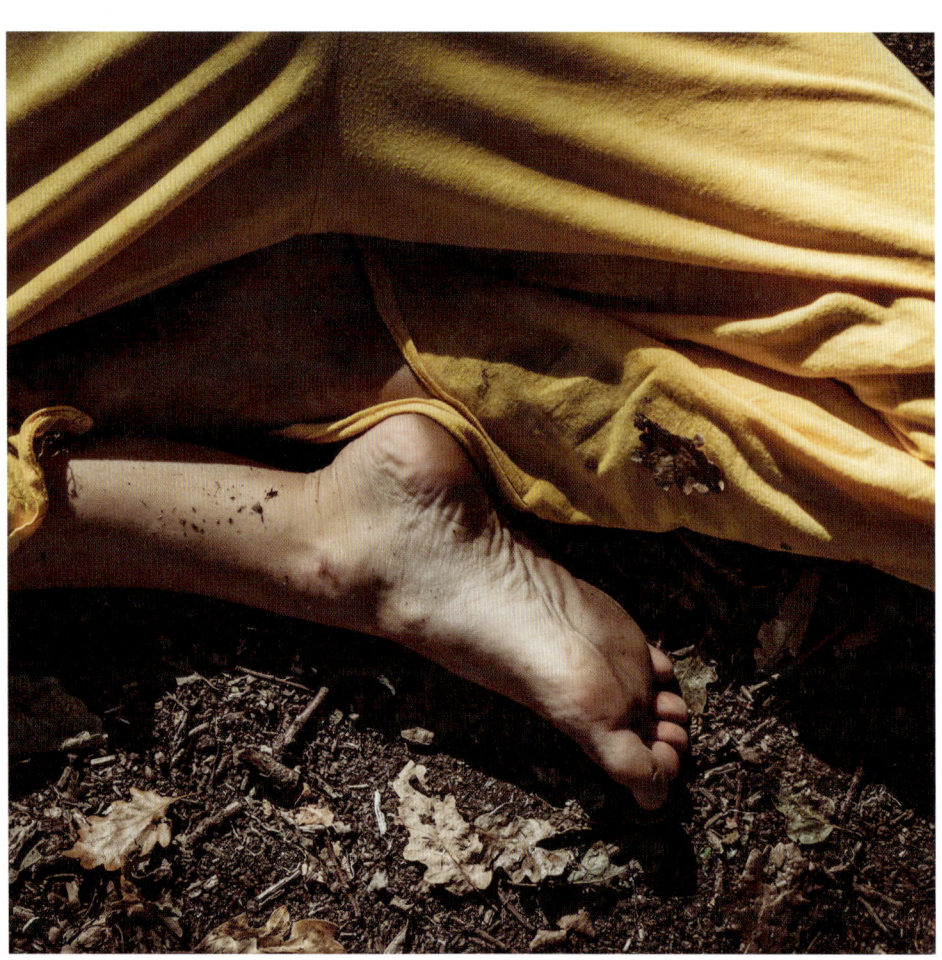

Process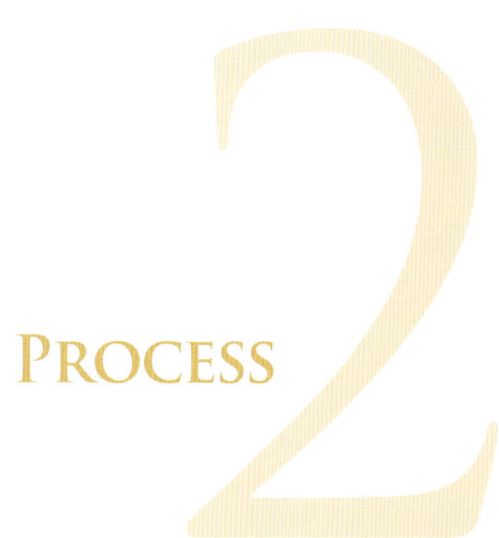

We process the past as it comes into the foreground of the present.

There are two realities: the reality of daily existence with its attendant consciousness and the reality that transcends it. We suspend familiar experience for short periods and discover there is more going on beneath the surface. Change is a process yielding the tension of well-molded patterns. Embedded memories often surface. Vivid recollections may emerge in tandem with realization and insight. Bringing the past to light is not an intention but an accepted aspect of deeper group work. Bygone events and the feelings around them are easily revealed.

Consciousness can be more powerful than the experiences it has absorbed regardless of their content. Insight arises from the space beneath personal history and may emerge on the back of re-experiencing past events. The preconscious, subconscious, and possibly unconscious aspects of 'one consciousness' (see Chapter 4 for Freud's divisions of consciousness) may open to a penetrating, lucid, dynamized consciousness that draws past experiences to the surface of the mind. We are our own therapists. The word therapy is derived from the Greek *therapeia,* meaning attendant. We listen to ourselves and attend to what we notice.

Awakening consciousness awakens the history enfolded within it. We do not invite these experiences or begin sessions with the idea of illuminating past events. Anything that arises does so without prior suggestion, but if people refer to memories the process is worth acknowledging. Shedding old stuff is healthy and transformative. Some memories may be poignant, and students can have profound experiences during class work. Other experiences may concern a time when childhood consciousness was passing through an impressionable stage, such as the lucid recollection of an aunt's arrival, an adult's face, or the feeling of a specific day. Many students quietly access memories and have illuminating insights about life. Yet others may have significant dreams and experience noticeable shifts in internal behavior. Students may wish to share memories there and then, or discuss them following class work, or let them settle, perhaps to share them another time.

Conditioning can inhibit or be selective with memory. An experience made present may be emotionally charged, but as often as not is simply *seen*. Lucid consciousness

Chapter 2

can dissolve the emotion associated with the memory as it surfaces. It is accepted that the upper levels of the brain can inhibit the lower and older parts responsible for emotion and memory. When we are free from mental content and the "brakes come off," we *awaken* to past experiences in the present. We do not revert *to* the past. Intensive consciousness draws the past *into* the now. The past comes forward and is processed by the clarity of consciousness in the present.

> "Last Tuesday something moved deeply in me. When we were laying down and I was opening my heart to the universe with your guidance I felt asleep but awake. I entered into a vision of my own life which has been very painful for some time. But this time wasn't – I didn't resist the journey, it all happened before my mind interfered, I guess.
> I was abused by my cousin when I was seven or eight years old and that image came very clearly in that vision on Tuesday. The vision/dream was very real and it was not like I remember it but a different 'view of the same moment,' like as if the camera was placed in a different angle of the room. It was not painful to witness, it did not bring any emotion, I was just observing it. The vision/dream was intense but short.

> When I finished the session with you I sat in my Shala quiet, and I began to cry deeply, and again for not very long, but it came from a deep place in me and then finished. I felt I have finally entered into a healing space, I thought I had before but I didn't know what my heart was keeping there, kind of hiding it from my memories of a scared child." *(The experience of a Yoga teacher having participated in an online two-hour workshop)*

Whatever their nature, emergent experiences are a consequence of our tendency for expansion:

It is the correlative movement of organic expansion or contraction that is the real generator of the language of the emotions. (Fouillée 1887)

> "I get very different things from each year and can see how the progression is so unbelievably powerful in deepening my experience and understanding. Just when I think I've 'got' something, I immediately realize it's another layer and there is layer upon layer upon layer – never ending. To feel it bodily, emotionally, and spiritually is awe inspiring, challenging, and reassuring – all at once." *(Nadine, Birth Educator, What Lies Beneath (WLB) course)*

Anchors

A clear sense of self supports the release of old patterns. Stability is provided by background tissue sensation acting as an anchor as the inner reaches of consciousness come to awareness. Neuroscientist Antonio Damasio writes: "It is intriguing to think that the constancy of the internal milieu is essential to maintain life and that it might be a blueprint and anchor for what will eventually become a self in the mind" (Damasio 2000). In other words, the physiology of sensation gives us a base. Stability also comes from combining attention with detachment. At some point the lucid intensity of consciousness may take over as a stabilizing force. Our presence also provides the trust needed for students to negotiate their experience. A stable, untainted presence lies beneath personal history, and its function is simply presence. Holding the space gives the stability and trust needed for people to move beyond themselves.

> "The last weekend was for me the most amazing yet. Something was released, to the extent of feeling quite emotional, and I'm still feeling the benefit. Even my face feels different, wide open with an urge to smile." *(Jane, Yoga Teacher, WLB Course)*

Dependency

Good and sometimes amazing experiences *(be amazed)* include feelings of love, joy, and an absence of anxiety, doubt, or defensive patterning and lead to a sense of freedom and unitive realization. The shyest individuals may come out of themselves. All concerned release the natural opiates (oxytocin and endorphins) that create a productive dependency between teacher and group.

This is a much less intense but similar hormonal release to the one that stimulates attachment and dependency following birth. "For a certain time following birth both mother and baby are impregnated with opiates (morphine like hormones and endorphins). Opiates induce states of dependency – an attachment will be likely to develop" (Odent 1999). The hormonal release in group work instills a dependency as the group associates the teacher with pleasant, enlightening feelings.

We also tune hormonally to the voice of others. Anatomical data suggests that the auditory system is mature in the middle of fetal life. If the voice is associated with pleasant sensations, we become more responsive and open up more readily to change. The effect of a teacher's voice may continue beyond class work. Biological scientist Rupert Sheldrake suggests "a law of contact." He writes: *"Things that have been in contact with each other continue to act on each other at a distance after the physical contact has been severed … separated parts that were once in contact remain linked to each other at a distance"* (Sheldrake 2011).

Dependency is initially productive as it assists the intention of the teacher. As the work continues, a nonattachment approach to the sensations and the outcome balances the level of dependency (*what will I do*

Chapter 2

when you go on a break?). Students learn to rely on the intensity of their own focus. This does not stop them coming back. They continue as participants, not as dependents. The relationship is similar to the traditional custom of a student attaching himself to a teacher or guru until his education is complete and guidance no longer needed. The practice of nonattachment began with what was considered an essential attachment.

Security

Definitions of *vulnerability* include *unguarded, exposed, unfortified,* and *resistless.* They are instrumental qualities in resolving ego supremacy and paving the way for transcendency and insight. Enabling and supporting these qualities requires an atmosphere of safety and trust. The teacher, the nature and pace of the work, and the surrounding environment should provide a feeling of security. Light humor (if it comes up), gentle focus, and ease of manner dissolve the tensions arising from potential insecurity. Above all, a teacher's integrity should be deliberately projected as a *feeling*.

Deep and sustained release of tension is effective on several levels. Tissues "move around," dormant memories surface, and snapshots of the past may come into focus. Broadly speaking and at each end of the spectrum, personal history reveals two kinds of people: those life pushes inward, who find it difficult to come out, and those life pulls outward, who cannot find their way back in. The most unlikely individuals find depth, and some you would expect to find expansion easily cannot, at least not for some time. We might over or underestimate students. It is sometimes best not to estimate! Estimation is not assessment based on time spent together. It is easy to read tensions, mechanical aspects, body types, and physical progress. But assessing how someone *is* requires a deeper intuition. This aspect unfolds naturally. We are not running encounter groups, although people will encounter themselves on some level. We might assess some people naturally, a symbiotic assessment, hardly knowing information has registered. Someone drawing our attention may be given additional security by addressing the group as a whole with him or her in mind.

Anxiety or unease can easily surface. The feeling that things are not as well as they could be may be disguised. The initial release of tension can evoke anxiety. This can be so commonplace it escapes awareness. Strong tension creates strong anxiety. Some people feel panic when they encounter resistance. An untoward background sense of anxiety provoked by gentle engagement may be a consequence of past experience. Entering the body unprepared, without calmness and with an agitated mind, sows the seeds for more unease. This kind of approach is relevant to our classes and courses. It recognizes an awareness considered necessary by other therapeutic approaches that address the human condition. It is too easy to get caught up in how to do postures, what should follow what, Sanskrit terminology, fascial elaboration, and Eastern philosophy. In the process we might overlook who we have in front of us: their insecurities, resistances, fixed ideas and frailties, and their experience!

Process

> "Like you said, the course 'shakes us up.' I am finding each weekend is going deeper. It's accumulative, getting stronger, but also I'm calmer. The last weekend I had the most amazing experience, feeling and clear seeing of being in the womb and of giving birth. It wasn't frightening at all. It was beautiful, peaceful, and healing. I felt it was me in the womb, reconnecting to myself the child within – perhaps also with parts that have got lost over the years. However, the births were the births of the two babies I lost in miscarriages. Having never given birth, it was a profound experience – one of great joy and healing. Although we think we have healed there is always some part that needs a little more. However, I felt that this was healing and a rebirth, of giving life spiritually. It touched my heart and brought the most amazing colours which spread throughout my body." *(Helen, Yoga Teacher, WLB course)*

The past unfolds into the present. The space of the present receives past experiences as if they are new experiences. The movement of the present *sees*, highlights, and releases, unresolved experiences and significant memories.

Coming out

As we bring people (and ourselves) out of positions we bring with us the mental and emotional space that has opened out. It is important how we *come out*. We should return slowly and in a considered manner, so as not to fill the creative space with extraneous activity. Realizations may continue as we change position. On a physical level we may come out of expansion but on other levels are still in expansion. The ego can attempt to re-establish its grip and fill the newfound space before the group has had time to adjust to where it has been, and still may be. As we *come out,* the group see one another again. Engaging with other faces stimulates the ego and inhibits the group field. We should re-engage with others slowly, at first keeping the eyes down, soft gazing toward the floor. Waiting enhances assimilation, before moving on to another stage or changing position.

Lynne McTaggart refers to a group coming out of deep meditation:

They were exhausted when they'd finished, overwhelmed by a kind of sensory overload when they returned to the here and now. It was as though they'd entered into some super consciousness, and once they'd come out of it, the world was more intense. The sky was bluer, sounds were louder, everything more deliciously real. It was if, in tuning into those barely perceptible signals their senses had been turned to maximum. Once they re-joined the world, ordinary volume bombarded them with sight and sound. (McTaggart 2003)

Our students are unlikely to be exhausted. If anything they may be *spaced* out, and also stimulated. But Lynne McTaggart's observation resonates. Resurfacing while having transcended conditioned limitations of consciousness needs time for processing. We are returning to the so-called normal world in

Chapter 2

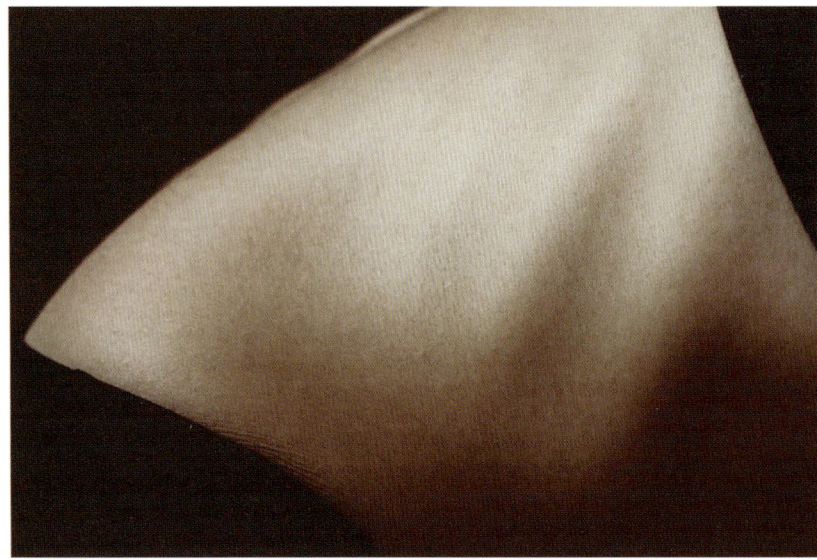

The past unfolds into the present. The space of the present receives past experiences as if they are new experiences. The movement of the present sees and releases unresolved experiences and significant memories.

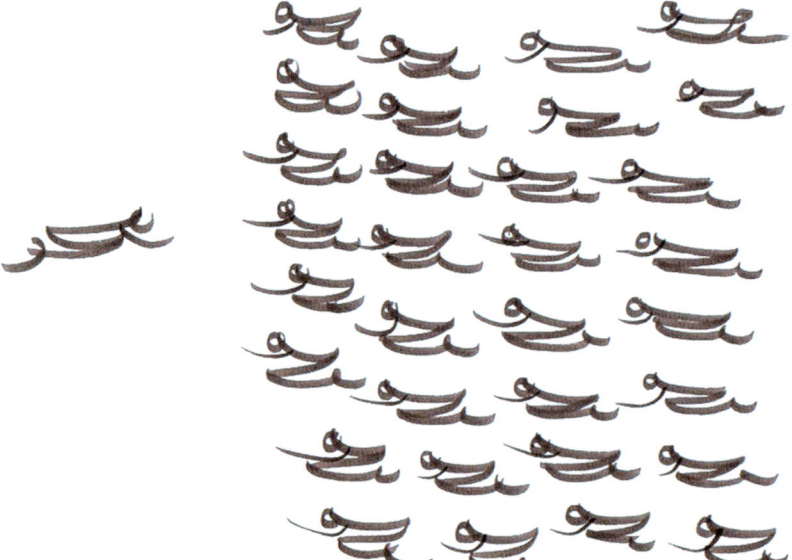

We should re-engage with others slowly, at first keeping the eyes down, softly gazing toward the floor. Waiting enhances assimilation.

an alternative state. Acknowledging the shift enables consciousness to adjust to deeper levels. Transitioning from one way of being to another is profound. A measured recognition and acknowledgment of *how we are* assists the ego in assimilating the changes. On the other hand, excessive analysis may inhibit further change, and we should try to keep things soft and light in appreciation of the feeling in the room.

PROCESS

> "Course doesn't seem the right word. I feel that is the point. The experience can't for me be put into words. But my understanding of myself and my place in the world has grown immeasurably. In my view it is your giving of yourself that has helped this growth ... the personal experiences and anecdotes." *(Steve, Yoga Teacher, WLB Course)*

A teacher's process: exposure and creative doubt

Creative insight is founded on a continuous movement of insightfulness. We expose our understanding there and then, as it emerges. In exposing our moment-to-moment experience we expose ourselves. There is no supportive formula or time to work it out. The immediacy and honesty of the experience provide the basis for transformational work. Sensing this, students have the trust to join us in current experience. Exposing ourselves enhances the quality of the work. The word *courage* comes from the Latin *cor* meaning *heart*, and in the ordinary sense *bravery. All senses of the word stem from the notion that the heart is the centre of feeling, thought and character* (Chambers Dictionary of Etymology). If we are not to "control" groups, we need the emotional flexibility to intuit and negotiate with the flow of change and teach from the heart.

What do we expose? Our ongoing experience, our nowness, our personal space, depth, sense of wonder and amazement (the smile), our vulnerability and heightened understanding, our insight and *knowing*, and perhaps our unsentimental love. We cannot expose insight without exposing ourselves. Realization is not selective. Students need to trust us but we must trust ourselves, our perceptions, and the work we have invested in. The energy of authentic teaching is released by exposure. Hesitate when expedient, but also trust what comes and go with the sense of it as it arises. Trusting authentic wisdom is a part of a teacher's process.

Sharing our experience enhances our guidance and its impact. Holding the space while being open to our experience brings extraordinary depth and a spontaneous quality to the work. Accepting a deeper calm, slowing down perception and response, sensing tissue reorganization, and acknowledging the release of our conditioning and a need for emotional stability are instrumental factors in doing our job. The more we take part in the process, the more powerful the process becomes. Accepting our vulnerability is not emotional lability but a willingness to show ourselves in the light of transformative experience. Our authority is tempered by *knowing nothing in particular* and staying in the present without prior knowledge (although we may call on it). Previous discoveries inhibit current insight. The guiding principle is right-now wakefulness at the time of delivery.

A sense of self holds the group but differs from confidence. Confidence based on past experience is limited, heavy, and inhibits creativity. Past experience is necessary for holding a group in their exploration, but we cannot be confident about the unknown. In this respect confidence closes us down. Venturing into unknown territory involves uncertainty and a sense of vulnerability supported by a present sense of self.

Chapter 2

Authenticity involves opening the heart and going beneath the mask of yoga teacher. Vulnerability and tenderness awaken creativity. The skill is to hold a group in its depth while being in ours. We transcend our habitual mind as our ego guides others. If we feel that we are taking a chance, we are learning to trust insightfulness. The word *doubt* comes from the Latin word *dubitare* meaning *to hesitate* or *waver in opinion*. Creative hesitation and doubt tempers insight and is productive. Creative doubt may arise when we are deeply engaged and beyond the constraints of familiarity. It compels us to trust current perception, consider our words, and have faith in a group's ability to convert our guidance into their experience. Creative doubt questions the quality of the process in order to give the best possible experience for others.

Processing is assisted by spotlighting the relationship between consciousness and the tissues. *The conditioned mind* displays an ever-changing chaos of thoughts and feelings that rearrange themselves in response to the magnification of the experience. *The conditioned body* continually reorganizes itself in response to a sensory awakening. As mind and body change, they inform and modify each other. A newfound sense of freedom releases the ego into the unknown. We can describe new experiences as we experience them. There are those who transform there and then and those who need more time. Once a little hesitation has done its job, we can project our understanding. Its effect can exceed expectations.

Stage fright

In the beginning, and sometimes beyond the beginning (of teaching) particularly with new groups, there may be a little stage fright, something that is common to seasoned actors in spite of their experience. Philosopher William James had this to say:

"Stage-fright" is the only extreme degree of that wholly irrational personal self-consciousness which everyone gets in some measure, as soon as he feels the eyes of a number of strangers fixed upon him, even though he be inwardly convinced that their feeling towards him is of no practical account. This being so, it is not surprising that the additional persuasion that my fellow-man's attitude means either well or ill for me, should awaken stronger emotions still. (James 1884)

As we temper wide-ranging aspects of behavior and bring them into a field of equanimity, we cannot know the minds or opinions of others. If you are a little nervous on occasion, you are not alone. Teachers, some of long standing, have *moments*. Such *moments* are productive. They invite us to pause, become more considered, and draw us back to the flow of the present.

This is not the vulnerability of exposing creative insight. It is simply feeling nervous, for whatever reason. If needed, support comes from various sources. Touching on anatomy or the philosophy of others can be supportive. The mild physical resistance of a position, or giving our weight to the ground, gives us a base to return to. The deepest support comes from faith in our own experience. The unknown may be supportive because there is no content to be uncertain of. We guide others from emptiness. Emptiness has no uncertainty or certainty. When we find ourselves in unknown territory, we are where we should be.

Process

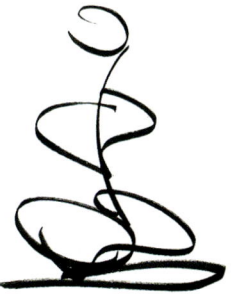

Teachers of long standing may have "moments."

When the work is done, when it has gone and familiarity returns, we may sometimes feel we could have done a better job. This is because it is over and we have discharged our creative energy. These feelings indicate that creativity does not run in straight lines. New experiences inform us and then assimilate into familiar patterning. More space is made available for receiving inspired and prolific insight the next time around.

"The realizations haven't stopped since the one I spoke about that happened during Friday's work. They seem so deep and complex it's hard to put them into words and even when I do the words don't do justice to the depth of them. My whole life is unravelling – seeing the masks that have been put on top of the actual deeply held beliefs, and so it's undoing both so I am in a place of neither, which feels amazingly free. I do know some of these have been there since birth and before that – actually have come in from a specific past life." *(Sue, Yoga Teacher, WLB course)*

Reaching out from experience

Group work is a cocreative process in progress requiring focused attention and an ever-clearing consciousness. Creativity manifests as we transcend tension and fuse into a *knowing*. Passing through gentle engagement, tuning in to the unpredictable behavior of tissue and the mind produces insightful realization. It takes faith to create from current experience without recourse to a method. "How to do" plays a role but is limited and it holds us back. When we allow the unknown to take over, egos yield and we find the language for describing newly discovered experience *as it arrives*. We reach out to others from current experience.

The privacy of thought and feeling is connected to a shared field. Each private mind confronts itself in the company of others engaged in the same process. We delve into ourselves with those we know, and often with those we don't. The experience is never the same, each time we start again. We provide the setting for yet to be discovered experiences. The unknown is a theater of space inviting creative sensation, consciousness, and insight. The theater does not change but its productivity does.

It seems to me

Teachers, speakers, and writers often use the term *it seems to me,* confirming that they speak from their own experience without external validation. This is the point: it is our own experience. *Knowing* is expressed through personal consciousness and forms the basis for wisdom and insight. *Knowing* is an aspect of consciousness underlying all that we are and do, with others or alone. Whatever comes our way, we learn to trust

Chapter 2

and believe our own experience. How does it *seem to you*, and to what extent do you use how *it seems to you* when teaching others?

Many books on spiritual values, particularly by Eastern teachers, are without references or bibliography. Krishnamurti, Rajneesh, Iyengar, and others give few, if any, references to support their point of view and way of thinking. Aldous Huxley's enlightened foreword for *The First and Last Freedom* points out that Krishnamurti, wary of distractions, neither consulted nor referenced other minds. His message was based on an indelible faith in his experience. The best-selling book of all time, the Bible, brimming with insight, wisdom, understanding, and an abiding reverence for the unknown lacks a bibliography.

Faith in our own insight sustains a group. Supportive resources and initial guides are secondary to current inspiration and intuition. The process of a teacher and his or her students is ongoing. It begins during sessions and continues between sessions. An awareness prevails within and beyond our community, indicating that things are changing.

> "The cumulative effect of these last five weekends has been quite profound for me. It feels like it has really accelerated an unwinding process that I feel like I've been in. We are continuously shedding and becoming, moving into deeper states of awareness and presence, letting go of habits and patterns that no longer serve us so we can emerge as the part of us who knows exactly how to be and how to become (like the embryo we sprouted from and continue to morph into), so we can soften and find freedom from the things which keep us in that gripping, contracted state, so we can heal and make whole again." *(Stephanie, Yoga Teacher, WLB course)*

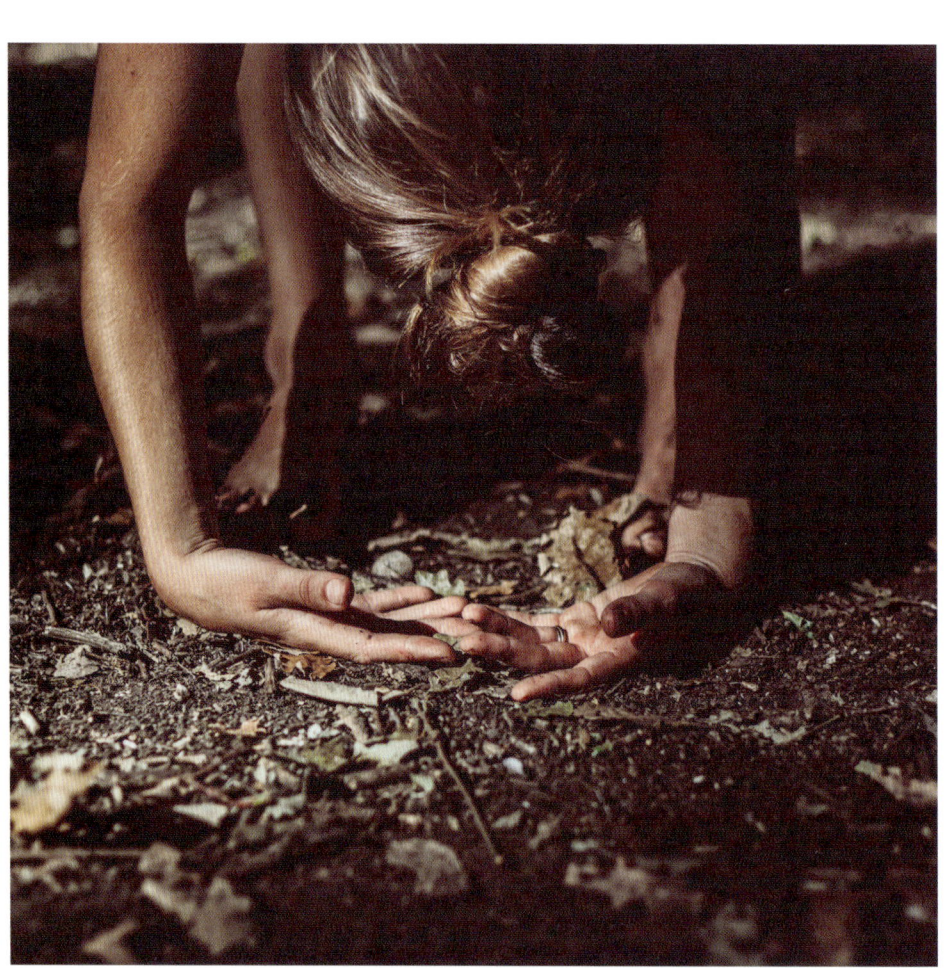

Embodiment 3

The deeper we go, the less we find. Reorganization takes place on another level.

Our minds are embodied and our bodies are known to our minds: we embody ourselves. To *embody* means *to give human shape to, to personify*. Our bodies reflect our practice but other relevant qualities of practice are without physical substance. Nonmaterial qualities arise from a material base, and have more power than the physical substance that produces and supports them.

The qualities we seek arise from a physical sense of self. We would be unlikely to find presence, lucidity, calmness, and respect without a body to house them. We have also embodied the conditioning that inhibits the expression of finer qualities. Many people, to a greater or lesser extent, are *unembodied* with a disconnect between psyche and soma. An exaggerated example might be Alexander Lowen's observation that the loss of identity of the ego with the body is the central crisis in schizophrenia (Juhan 1987).

Yoga's nonmaterial reality is an internal quality that is unveiled by practice, experienced inwardly, and expressed outwardly as alternative conduct. Embodied yoga might be an emotion underlying all other emotion, in that it emotes (moves out) from within as an expressive quality.

As our minds enter our bodies are we or our students embodying the more positive states of mind? Entering the body with a conditioned mind may reinforce some aspects of conditioning. Ideally, we should enter the body with a quality of mind we aspire to. A teacher's conditioned mind may enter the bodies of others and sow the seeds of conditioned yoga. Positive qualities are usually, but not always, embodied from the start.

Consciousness: the common denominator

If we embody anything, it is consciousness. For us consciousness refers to a quality beyond normal wakeful alertness. Eastern traditions recognize the importance of awakening consciousness as the ground of being. We are the embodiment of consciousness. Bodies may differ but consciousness has no definitive margins. The depth and expansiveness of consciousness may differ between individuals but its potential for unlimited

Chapter 3

space remains the same. This potential has given mysticism the idea that consciousness preceded the body, and we have evolved from cosmic consciousness.

The Western view proposes that consciousness has arisen from the body. Neuroscientist Antonio Damasio in his book, *The Feeling of What Happens*, suggests that for consciousness to have evolved it had to be reflected back to itself. Consciousness needs an object of reflection, such as internal activity, soft tissue sensation, mental activity, or a response to an external object (hence an object of meditation). The sensation of living tissue has provided an ideal reflector for the evolution of consciousness. Damasio (2000) proposes the following:

- Basic consciousness, the forerunner of consciousness as we know it, is stimulated by older areas of the brain, from the brain stem upward into the sensory areas of the cerebral cortex.

- Neural and chemical routes from the body to the brain suggest the body influenced the evolution of consciousness via the brain.

- Primitive sensory structures involved in gravitational, proprioceptive, interoceptive, and kinesthetic senses were involved in an evolving consciousness.

In other words, the evolution of consciousness, and present-day consciousness, has been and is still stimulated by the senses, notably by proprioceptive and kinesthetic

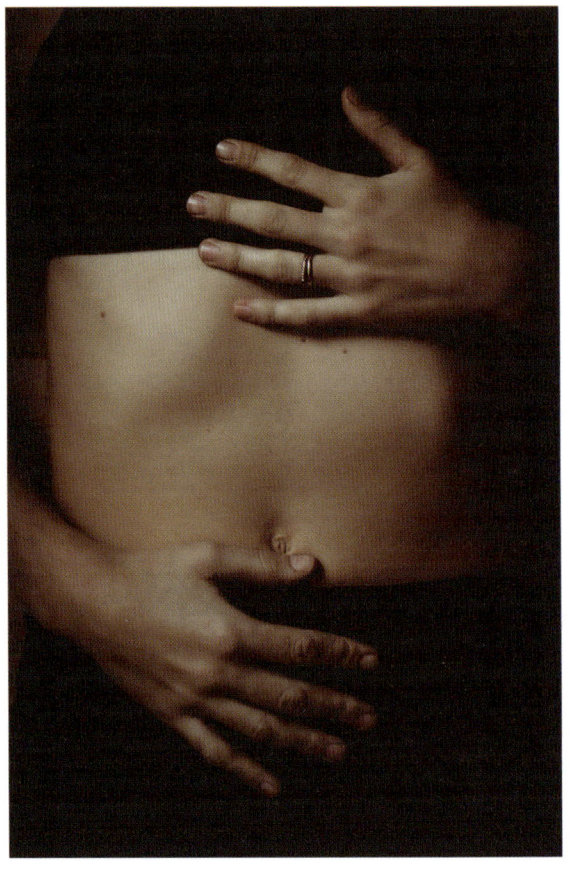

Living tissue provided the ideal reflector for the evolution of consciousness.

sensation from the musculoskeletal system in association with incoming signals from the environment. Consciousness arose from, and is enhanced by, physical sensation and sensory perception. Consciousness changes as it senses the body. Our sense of self comes from our bodies and our minds, providing a foundation for the yoga experience. A self has a plasticity amenable to change, the degree of which depends upon the grip of the conditioning.

EMBODIMENT

Damasio states:

I advanced the possibility that the part of the mind we call self was, biologically speaking, grounded on a collection of nonconscious neural patterns standing for the part of the organism we call the body proper ... the brain reconstructs the sense of self moment by moment. We do not have a self sculpted in stone and, like stone, resistant to the ravages of time. Our sense of self is a state of the organism. (Damasio 2000)

Depth, embodiment, and sensation

We can sense the depth of embodiment on several levels:

- Material depth involves a myriad of tissue sensations, fluid rhythms, and respiratory movements. Depth can be felt within the fabric of the tissues.

- Nonmaterial depth presents as a sense of space within consciousness.

- A deep *unitive* awareness includes everything within the field of consciousness. In the process of deepening physical experience and spatial consciousness we deepen the sense of unitive awareness.

Sensation and consciousness awaken together. We awaken ourselves as we awaken a deeper tissue sensitivity. Sentient consciousness arises from awakening sensory physiology. Total experience stems from the embodiment of consciousness. Damasio suggests: "it is possible that feelings are poised at the very threshold that separates being from knowing and thus have a privileged connection to consciousness" (Damasio 2000).

Body awareness and mind awareness belong to consciousness. The quality of consciousness is enhanced by refining our ability to sense our tissues. We do not possess consciousness. We *are* consciousness. Awareness moves between sensation, mental content, and consciousness itself. Consciousness is dynamic and we can dynamize it further by being attentive to its presence. When we direct consciousness we discover its potential for piercing the sleep of conditioning.

Consciousness is our common denominator. Regardless of physical ability, consciousness has vast possibilities. Although the body has limitations, we can begin to understand the profoundness of consciousness by engaging with the soft tissues, regardless of postural accomplishment. The body is a door to an alternative way of being. Going inward takes us closer to our true nature by dissolving past experience that clings to the outer layers of behavior.

We meet the external environment through skin and surface connective tissue, the interface between the inner and outer worlds. Deep connective tissue lining the cavities, surrounding the bones, investing the heart and diaphragm is continuous with the surface of the body, which in turn is emotionally and spiritually continuous with the ego and with primary consciousness.

Chapter 3

> Draw students into ever-deepening sensations – not so much as to lock them down but not so little that they lack engagement. Slowly and calmly release your sensitivity and notice what "happens." Take the group with you. See what comes to mind as you open together.

Embodied authenticity

Working through patterns involves each person processing personal sensations. We arrive at a common experience by passing through differing intensities at different times. Entering ourselves can only be authentic. The immeasurable variations and intensities of human conditioning remind us that *the way in* is personal from moment to moment. Each of us is authentic. Given the same posture, breath, teacher, suggestion, and moment, each of us will respond authentically. No two people have the same timing, texture, response, or experience. Authenticity emerges as *we* enter into ourselves because we are conditioned in different ways and with different intensities. We become more alike as we reach and share deeper levels of experience.

Sages remind us that yoga is hidden beneath embodied conditioning waiting to reveal itself. Yoga, embodied from or before birth, represents our deepest aspect, an aspect that has accompanied and promoted our evolution. Yoga and consciousness unfold together but are mired in distraction along the way. Authenticity springs from the realization that no one can reveal yoga for us. Yoga and the depth of consciousness it reveals is an authentic experience. Only we can reclaim our essence.

We cannot measure the depth and scope of another's consciousness, nor measure our own. Consciousness is immeasurable and has unlimited potential. What are the benchmarks for progress? The term *enlightenment* lacks resonance through overuse. Many of us have enlightened moments or periods in our lives. Many people appear enlightened without knowing it. We all engage in the requisite superficiality of social life and formal communication. An awareness of what we say, how we act, and a sensitive appreciation of the totality of life distinguishes one person's consciousness from another's. Insight and a sense of realization, alongside physical ease, are indications that things are changing.

Depth of embodiment

Definitions of the word *depth* include: *profound*, *inmost part* and *penetration*. Mystics and yogis investigated their inmost experience by penetrating their conditioning and came to profound conclusions. They entered and observed their feelings, emotions, thoughts, and quality of consciousness. They practiced an ongoing inward movement intended to discover an alternative reality:

And yet and yet,
concealed in us is a sublime depth
we sense only dimly
but, when revealed, raises us
to undreamt heights
beyond all petty notions
of who we are.
That depth is our unblemished future.
(Lalla in Feuerstein 1997)

Embodiment

The deeper we go, the closer we become as we pass through individual conditioning. We meet within the depth of consciousness. We become depth's congregation coming together in an unknown place. Life begins *in* depth. Implantation occurs within the deepest recesses of the body. Embryonic activity unfolds from a deep center. The skin, our encapsulating membrane, unfolds from the deepest and earliest layers of tissue.

Depth begins with the sensation of tissue responding and moving. Depth also has various contributors. Life experience, an interest in the nature of experiencing, and a reflective, contemplative mind coalesce to give the sense of a deeper self. A tendency to think and feel deeply may be more pronounced in some than others, but everyone has the potential for deepening their awareness. We might be emotionally, intellectually, or spiritually deep. We can have deep thoughts, be deep in thought, or immerse in deep mindfulness or meaningfulness. We can relate deeply, love deeply, and be deeply in love. Depth comes to light by being drawn inward *by* something.

The deeper mind is a feeling, a presence, a deeper sense of self. Georg Feuerstein describes the depth mind as "the activator," a place where the residue of all activity is deposited, a place of deep agitation. The deeper layers of consciousness hold memories of early socialization and conditioning no longer needed by awareness and stores the psychic residue of one's actions and experiences that color behavior (Feuerstein 1992). Beneath these layers exists a mind of undisturbed composure. The *deeper* mind enjoys space and freedom from past influences. Sinking our awareness to deeper levels clears old experiences and provides fertile territory for the emergence of personal insight and wisdom.

Yoga suggests we can transcend (as opposed to analyze) preconscious material released into consciousness. The traditional approach focused relentlessly on loosening the ego self and breaking through repressed material that inhibited growth. This was and is achieved by disidentification, i.e., witnessing unwanted material without attachment. Depth is a quality. We feel its power in practice and use its presence to hold groups in their attention.

Deepening

Deepening sensation does not guarantee deepening consciousness. Noticing the mind's interference in tandem with deep sensory inquiry enables old material to surface and dissolve and allows uncluttered consciousness to emerge. Thought and analysis permeate the upper layers of consciousness. Pure depth is beyond thought. Some traditional yogis suggested a depth beyond experience, suggesting that all experience was at odds with our true nature. The value of this is debatable. It borders on trance. Pure consciousness has a crystal clear awareness of the totality of life. Conscious experience is the pinnacle of human evolution but with a sting in the tail. Consciousness has become clogged with unnecessary activity. For some practitioners it may be sufficient to soften the edges of habitual patterns, if not partially dissolve them. Anything beyond this leads to more transformative ways of being and requires sustaining deeper work.

Chapter 3

Deep body awareness deepens presence. Deep sensation is the physical representative of the deeper self. Likewise, depth of presence deepens attention and therefore body awareness. Awakening consciousness through sensation involves intense focus on surface tissue. Focusing on the body surface needs deeply focused attention because it holds the potential distraction of resistance. Awakening the skin and superficial fascia can be as, if not more, profound as awakening the spine. Embryonic surface tissue unfolds from the deep tissue investing the embryo's primitive spinal cord and brain. Surface sensation is an essential aspect of the central nervous system.

Physical experience gives us a base. We move from sensation into nonmaterial realization and return to sensation as and when necessary. Sensation is not the whole thing. Deepening does not stop at a specified place. Consciousness continues to deepen as it feeds from sensory experience.

Creative engagement

Creative engagement teaches us:

- that consciousness is embodied
- that sensory lucidity enhances lucid consciousness
- that consciousness opens in response to a release of physical tension
- that tissue engagement should be appropriate for revealing lucid consciousness
- about noticing the quality of internal behavior.

Tissue engagement gives us a material focus and invites inner space. Areas of recurrent, less yielding resistance are usually habituated and linked to other aspects of experience. They can be considered as local dysfunctions having an overall effect. As areas soften and open, the effect on internal behavior can be profound. Sensory changes and insight spring from the same source. The deeper and more expansive the sensation, the more profound the insight. As we slow down, pass through anatomy, and dissolve ideas on how we should be working, we can discover the finer sensations and notice their effect in time to make choices. Choosing a quieter attitude is essential for a seamless flow of sensation and consciousness.

Physical depth feels as if we are touching and being touched by a profound communication with the tissues. Moving inward draws our attention to anatomical features and their relationship. We may refer to spinal curves, pelvic and shoulder girdles, the sensitivity of nerves, and the nature of living tissue. We may acknowledge the fascial web, the relationship between the skin and deep tissue, respiratory dynamics, or the benefits of visualizing and sensing the heart.

Deeper sensations take us into and beyond the habitual mind, and we may notice agitation, anxiety, restlessness, timidity, self-esteem, excitement, or joy. We can be attentive to surface tissue while registering the ever-changing experience of us, in all its shades and irregularities. We may address the changing nature of sensation, but a conditioned free consciousness requires particular vigilance.

EMBODIMENT

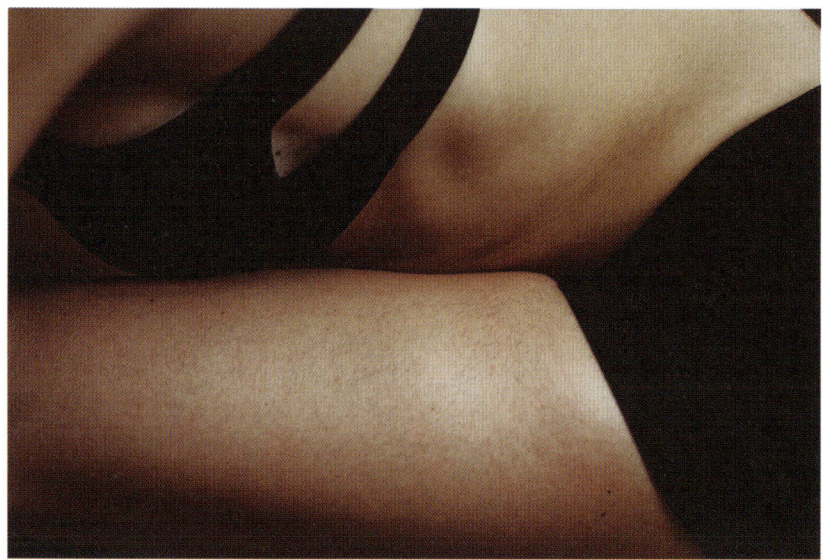

Dynamic consciousness dissolves conditioning.

Ultimate embodiment

An ultimate experience is not dependent on flexibility; if it were, Craniosacral Therapy would only benefit bendy people. The tantric tradition favored ecstatic experience by passing through sensation into more exquisite sensation. Transcendence goes into and through the object of transcendence and disperses it. We need sensation to transcend sensation. Expansion is neither an act of will or a deliberate separation of parts. Expansion is a pleasurable, involuntary expression of life and a tendency for tissue, and the energy that binds it, to radiate in all directions. Penetrating physiological engagement, and awakening expansion, dissolves conditioning and dynamizes consciousness.

Engaging the tissues directly may be outside the sphere of biomechanics, although we should consider mechanics and alignment. If necessary this can be addressed by positioning body parts accordingly and extending *toward the center* while focusing on given areas of engagement . The real work is the simple act of being attentive to consciousness entering tissue and tissue reflecting back to consciousness.

Dropping down

The roots of our self extend deeply down into sensory tissue and an ancient consciousness. To what extent can the roots be felt and how can they be found and revealed? Advanced practice implies depth of sensation, depth of being, depth of understanding, and depth of presence. We can drop down softly into ourselves, move our attention beyond anatomical reference, and follow an inward and downward movement of consciousness. The upper reaches sink quietly into the lower reaches, transforming practice and teaching.

Chapter 3

Pass through an area of gentle engagement while remaining empty. Drop quietly and softly into your deepest places. Stay there while observing the mental and physical changes. Invite others to join you.

We can go into the body and make up our own minds. Once we have established consciousness as the companion of sensation we can take a closer look.

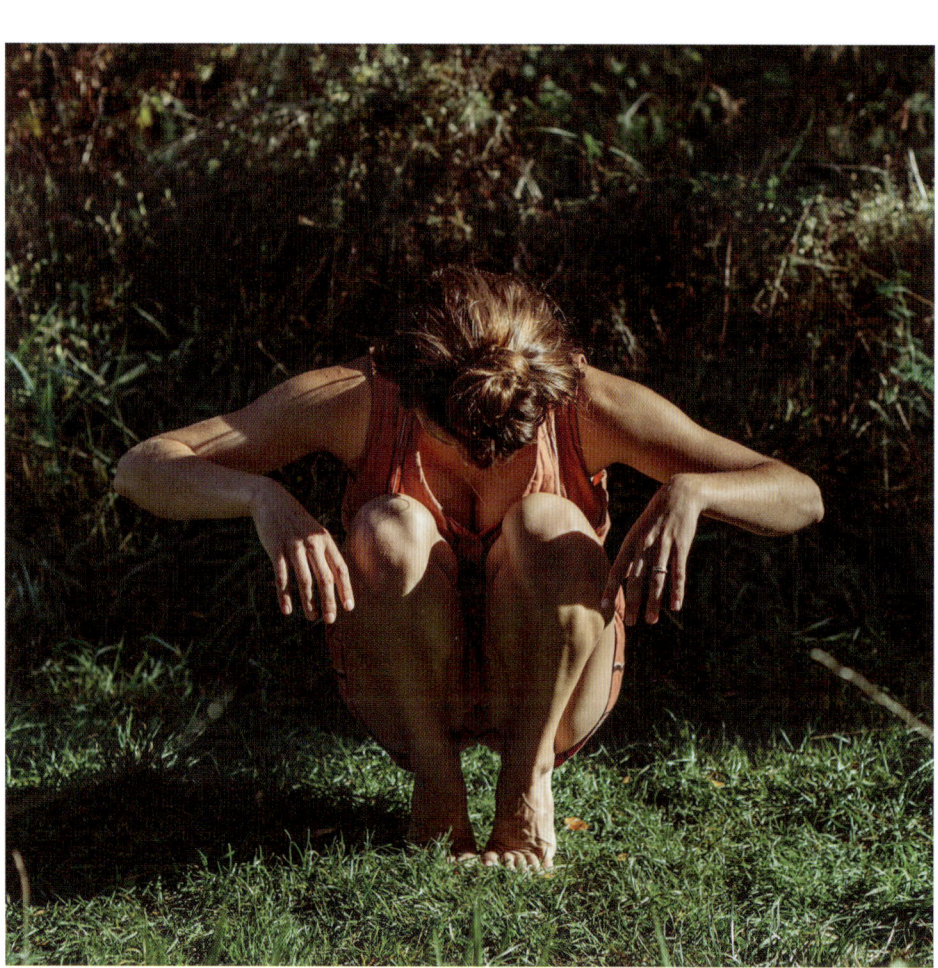

DIVIDING THE INDIVISIBLE 4

We cannot help but be students of consciousness. The mind is ever present, rarely switching itself off, and should it decide to do so it lacks the means. The body invites depth and expansion, consciousness even more so.

Given the body you have, if offered the choice between an ability to perfect every known posture, or maintain your current practice and have peace of mind and lucidity for the rest of your days, how would you choose? The former does not guarantee the latter. We are attracted to the scope of physical sensation, but consciousness, given its unpredictability and potential, may be more intriguing. The mind can go anywhere it wishes, it can disturb itself, observe itself, or leave itself alone. The body is earthbound. Consciousness can play between the stars.

The body-self is not an inviolable stronghold against the corrosion of ontological doubts and uncertainties: it is not in itself a bulwark against psychosis.

—R. D. Laing (1960/2010)

R. D. Laing acknowledges that attending to the body, without attending to the mind, consciousness, and feelings, does not go far enough in addressing psychoemotional disturbance and conflict. Laing's groundbreaking book on schizophrenia, *The Divided Self*, attracted many who recognized his insight as an essential contribution to the humanistic movement of the 1960s (Laing 1960/2010).

Have you noticed the majority of us, yoga teachers included, are mildly or otherwise, bipolar, intermittently psychotic, quietly schizophrenic, unknowingly or knowingly neurotic, or simply anxious? Mental and emotional conflict is common to the human condition. Our minds are subject to the contagion of conditioning. This observation, made many centuries ago, led to the development of yoga and its interest in the nature of consciousness and the conditioned mind.

The body houses consciousness and the mind. Consciousness implies so much more than being conscious. Consciousness is more expansive than a mind or a self. In the strictest sense, consciousness and the mind are not synonymous. There is a distinction between the mind and consciousness. The mind is

Chapter 4

within consciousness. Consciousness is the process through which a mind can refer to itself. Yoga's interpretation of consciousness refers to an experience that includes deep awakening, expansion, lucidity, and dynamization. The mind is a part of consciousness and can focus on consciousness in order to change itself. Lucid, awakened consciousness contains the same activity as normal consciousness but puts it in a transcendent perspective.

The space of lucid consciousness can take or leave the mind's contents. We experience the potential depth and breadth of consciousness within a setting of consciousness.

Yoga edits the contents of the mind within consciousness, inviting us to choose between negative and positive aspects and look at what is actually relevant within the hubris. We learn to recognize mental activity for what it is and, if necessary, modify or penetrate the behavior of thought. Consciously addressing consciousness makes space for incoming material. Mulling over mental activity can be fruitful or disturbing depending on how we perceive it.

Consciousness encompasses awareness and we are aware of consciousness. Awareness takes in all the activity within its field. Dynamic consciousness, on the other hand, has a penetrating intensity, an intensification of attention that passes through and beyond everything within its field.

Consciousness is grounded in the body. We need the body's material sense from which to examine the nonmateriality of consciousness. Tissue engagement gives consciousness a point of reference. As the tension of tissue engagement disperses, consciousness itself can dissolve thought and conditioning. Dispersing tissue engagement disperses the tension of thought. We can work with the body while enabling the essence of consciousness.

Each of us is in reality an abiding psychical entity far more extensive than he knows … The Self manifests through the organism; but there is always some part of the Self unmanifested; and always, as it seems, some power of organic expression held in abeyance or reserve. (James 1902/2018)

Dividing the indivisible

Antonio Damasio writes: "If 'self-consciousness' is taken to mean 'consciousness with a sense of self,' then all human consciousness is necessarily covered by the term—there is just no other kind of consciousness as far as I can see" (Damasio 2000). His statement is in accord with Krishnamurti's subjective observation that *there is only one consciousness.* Consciousness is a continuum from below up, from above down, from a periphery to a center, or from a center to a periphery.

Evolutionary phases of consciousness are indivisible, and they are enfolded within one another. Exactly when and how each phase came about is unknown. Ancient phases of consciousness may have had a greater time span than more recent ego consciousness. Consciousness has taken the

Dividing the indivisible

time it needed to get from then to now, but stems from the same origin. The chemistry of behavior applies to ancient and current consciousness.

To understand behavior and experience, consciousness has been divided into layers, depths, and qualities. How experience arrives into consciousness is unknown, maybe because, pathology and trauma aside, consciousness and experience are indivisible, each having contributed to the unfoldment of the other. We are conscious of our experience and we experience consciousness. Experiences have stimulated the development of consciousness, and subsequent stages of consciousness have refined experience.

Consciousness and experience have driven each other, but yoga practitioners, through mindful experimentation, have separated experience from consciousness. We can observe experience from a lucid consciousness, but this too is the experience of observing one's experience, that is unless we enter a trance state and are unable to record the experience.

It is suggested that sensory information entered a primitive nervous system and stimulated the onset of a primordial consciousness that established an early self. Early consciousness thrived on sensory experience. A mind developed as consciousness unfolded, both grounded in the material base of a brain, supported by the body. Nonmaterial consciousness emanates from the material density of a body and brain. Living tissue is the material aspect of a self.

Tissue gives us substance and although immeasurably expressive is limited in expression compared to our minds, which are fluid, unbounded, unpredictable, and give us considerable potential for change. Mind and consciousness lack substance but are substantially present. The yoga experience

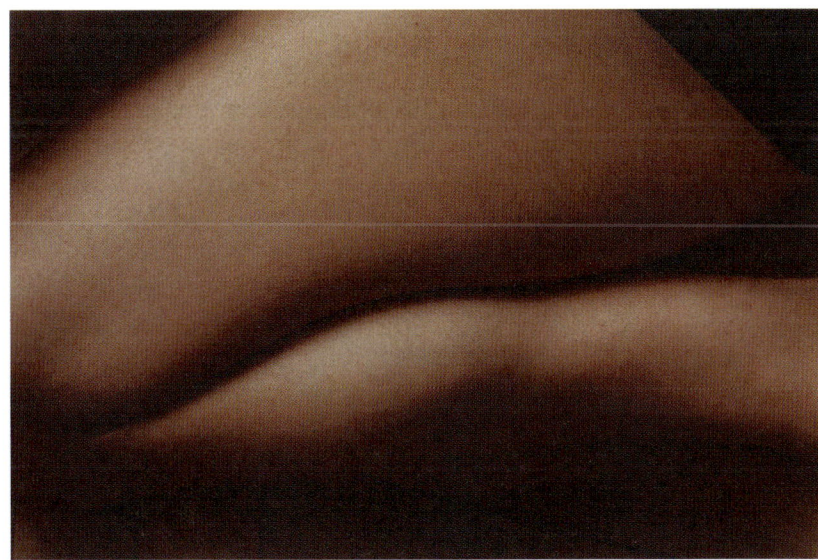

We can invite a less material body and a more material consciousness.

Chapter 4

invites a less material body and a more material consciousness. In tandem with physics, yoga proposes consciousness as a subtle form of matter and matter as a condensation of consciousness. Consciousness has a density that can be divided.

Ancient and recent aspects of consciousness influence each other. We bring the subconscious with us. Deeper experiences invite speculation as to what channels have opened up, or why they were previously inaccessible. Freud saw the difficulty in giving the mind an anatomical structural basis. The physical brain provides a mind, but the mind is without physical structure. An anatomy of the mind is contrived but provides a working framework.

Eastern practice identifies elements of consciousness on its own terms – an undertaking that spanned centuries of personal inquiry. In the West, the more recent advent of psychoanalysis, neuroscience, and physics have categorized elements of the mind and consciousness from a different though complementary perspective. Consciousness and minds are of the same fabric.

We could accept one consciousness containing variable *activity* and leave it at that. But the mind's drifting contents, its fixations, and the nature of consciousness present a variety of possibilities. Although seemingly indivisible, of the various elements identified some may be experienced. We are aware of consciousness, its contents, and aware of our material and nonmaterial self. We can also acknowledge various aspects of consciousness that have arisen out of sensation, out of one another, how they might resonate with our experience, and how their awakening contributes to our potential for change.

Dividing consciousness

Yoga suggests a consciousness beyond daily wakeful consciousness. Its totality is a force of nature. We have consciousness and consciousness has us. Consciousness can perceive itself in its raw state and we can use it to dissolve body–mind tension and conditioning.

According to Antonio Damasio, consciousness does depend most critically on brain regions that are evolutionarily older and are located in the depth of the brain rather than on its surface. The processes involved are anchored in ancient neural structures intimately associated with the regulation of life, rather than on the modern neural achievements of the neocortex which permit fine perception, language, and high reason. Consciousness arises from a deep and lower order. The light of consciousness is carefully hidden and venerably ancient (Damasio 2000).

The mind contains thought and consciousness contains the mind. Consciousness has involuntary roots. We didn't *do* consciousness for it to evolve, although our actions contributed to its development. At its simplest consciousness can be divided from below up into an unconscious, subconscious, preconscious, and conscious.

Consciousness unfolded into an awareness of itself. In *The Ever-Present Origin*, Jean Gebser goes further, proposing various evolutionary phases of consciousness and suggesting they remain latent in us. Each

DIVIDING THE INDIVISIBLE

phase is not superseded by the next but remains enfolded within its predecessors. The inception of each phase is imprecise, but each is a next stage emerging from our primal heritage. We bring all phases into present-day consciousness and may be aware of their presence during experiences encountered in practice. When we are *feeling* consciousness, what kind of consciousness might we be *feeling*?

Archaic consciousness

This suggests a total innocence that supports our sense of oneness with all things. It suggests a harmonious, undisturbed, nondifferentiated relationship with the universe preceding our awakening into conscious awareness (Gebser 1949/1985). Archaic consciousness may arise in advanced meditative states.

Magical consciousness

Magical consciousness reflects an egoless, boundless state, comparable to modern-day trance. Magical man acts without knowing but begins to experience himself as a part of a group having a profound unity with the world and wonder of it (Gebser 1949/1985). The "wonder" experience of magical consciousness is common in group work.

Mythical consciousness

This phase is still defined by group identity before the complete consolidation of the separate self. We step out of nature and begin to become conscious of our individuality. We no longer merge with the universe as we awaken to the beginning of a self and discriminate between our own experience and group experience. "Mythical consciousness indicates the onset of imagination, an awareness of inner life, and the polarity between group and separative consciousness. This phase mirrors the merging of group and personal experience" (Gebser 1949/1985). It is as if we touch mythical consciousness as we come out of the vast unitive feel, during deep-tissue meditative states, and discriminate between our own experience and that of the group.

Archaic, magical, and mythical consciousness continue to feed our experience. Oneness with the group blending with our individuality is the common experience.

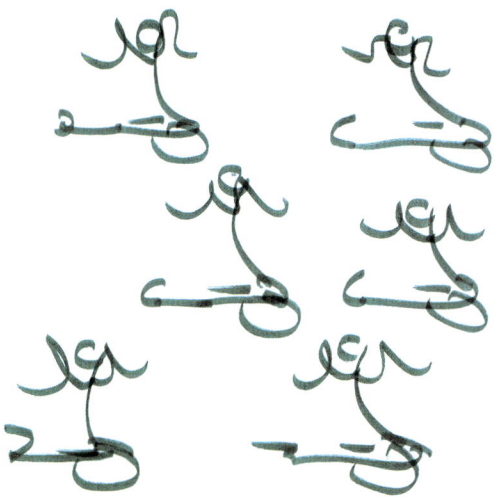

Archaic, magical, and mythical consciousness continue to feed our experience. Wonder, awakening, and oneness with the group are common experiences.

Chapter 4

Mental consciousness

Man leaves the protection of the group to further develop his individuality. Georg Feuerstein, paraphrasing Jean Gebser, describes this stage as becoming fully crystallized during the period around the eras of the Buddha, Lao Tzu, and Socrates. Man develops a dualistic, "either/or" consciousness, with a strong individualistic sense of identity. The separative ego is reinforced during the stage between mythical and mental consciousness. Logic emerged around this period (Feuerstein 1974). Mental consciousness may provide us with the tools needed to choreograph the group dynamic as we guide them through deeper states.

Our observations and suggestions to groups may spring from mental consciousness fed by the deeper realms of archaic, magical, and mythical consciousness.

Spatial consciousness

As we separated ourselves from our environment and the group, we moved into spatial consciousness, which we mastered through thought. Spatial consciousness gave us the inner space within which we could develop discursive thought (Gebser 1949/1985). Our work moves us between the presence and absence of thought, between inner space and the condensation of thinking. Spatial consciousness acts as the essential door to the yoga experience and how to communicate it.

We access spatial consciousness as we give space to our experience and give time for appropriate decision making in teaching. Our work highlights the benefits of spatial consciousness, while acknowledging a tendency for it to fill itself with activity of its own making.

Extended consciousness

Extended consciousness can cover a large area of the external environment and peer deeply into our internal environment (Gebser 1949/1985). Extended consciousness can blend our external and internal environment simultaneously. We can feel an inner depth connecting to the outer world. Tuning into this connection feels like the beginning of the combined microcosmic and macrocosmic experience. We tune into extended consciousness as we guide others through current experience and underlying depth, while drawing attention to the bigger picture.

Integral consciousness

Integral consciousness is a consolidation of consciousnesses that have unfolded from one another. Integral consciousness recognizes emotional fluency, personal responsiveness, reverence for all life, and the capacity for service and love. "We must submit to the difficult task of personally actualizing the essential features of the integral consciousness, such as self-knowledge, global thinking and social responsibility" (Feuerstein 1974).

Jean Gebser points out that *integral consciousness* is not identical to intelligence but is an *intensification* of consciousness rather than an expansion. Our work shows consciousness *intensification* as a consequence of the sensation of expansion. Sensory expansion illuminates consciousness as the central feature of our experience.

Gebser wrote: "There is no so-called unconscious. There are only various modalities (or intensities) of consciousness; a one-dimensional Magical, a two-dimensional Mythical and a three-dimensional Mental consciousness. And there will also be an integral four-dimensional consciousness of the whole" (Gebser 1949/1985). Perhaps we pass through all four dimensions.

Dynamic or pure consciousness

Dynamic or pure consciousness might be described as an awakened unification of all categories, characterised by lucidity, the feeling of oneness, and an advanced state of self-aware consciousness devoid of mental, emotional, or sensory distractions. Pure consciousness is a term used by Krishnamacharya as recounted by his son (Desikachar & Krusche 2014). But the term *dynamic* can be used in reference to pure consciousness due to its sheer force. Dynamic consciousness appears to cut through everything within its field of awareness including its concept of itself. The additional intensification of dynamic consciousness gives an impression of pervading all things.

Philosopher William James may have referred to dynamic consciousness when he wrote:

The fact is that mystical feeling of enlargement, union, and emancipation has no specific intellectual content of its own. ... as a rule, mystical states merely add supersensuous meaning to the ordinary outward data of consciousness. They are excitements like the emotions of love or ambition, [and they carry feelings] of vastness, of union, of safety, and of rest. (James 1902/2018)

Dynamic or pure consciousness *feels* as if it arises out of a spatial consciousness that gives space to everything within our experience. Spatial consciousness minimizes all experience within itself and produces a dynamically vital consciousness that cuts through all remaining activity. The result is a lucid force of emptiness, a powerfully flowing action without content or boundary.

Dynamic consciousness is the incisive tool that cuts through the walls of conditioning and leads to transcendent experiences. Words do not come easily at this point and come from a distance. We may deliver a well-spaced word or two to acknowledge the experience and anchor a group.

Rational consciousness

Georg Feuerstein observed that over the last several centuries consciousness has congealed and *rationalized*, a condition he describes as fatally imbalanced. We live by a rational consciousness which is deficient, corrupted (his perception), conditions our awareness, colors our perceptions, and is the antithesis of realization and the deeper yoga experience. Attending to rational consciousness, observing and penetrating its turbulence, is an essential aspect of our work.

Chapter 4

As we immerse with groups it seems clear that spatial consciousness provides an essential aspect of the entire experience. Space within consciousness, and space around conscious experience, enables a lucid appreciation of all that we are, do, and share.

> As sensation passes through awareness, look into your mind. Identify a spatial consciousness that contains your mind and is larger than the activity within it.

Minds

The terms mind and consciousness are interchangeable. The mind has been defined as the seat of consciousness, but consciousness represents the foundation for the mind. We refer to altered states of consciousness, not altered states of mind. We may have a state of mind in reference to mood, slant, or fixation. We might be in two minds or out of our minds.

As consciousness deepens and opens, it penetrates and opens the mind. Consciousness, the state of being aware, came first and is the medium through which we experience reality. The mind is the product of consciousness and is contained within the space of consciousness, and consciousness lies at the heart of the mind. The mind gives access to dynamic consciousness, and dynamic consciousness can penetrate the mind.

Consciousness is much more than our egos. It is even, according to yoga, much more than our minds. Scientists are beginning to ask the question, "How does mind give rise to consciousness?" Yoga would ask: "How does consciousness give rise to the mind?" (Iyengar 2005).

The mind is the tool of consciousness. We use our mind to turn our attention toward consciousness. The word *mind* comes from the old English word *gemynd* for memory, arising from the Greek *menos* meaning *intent* or *purpose*, a derivative of *mimneskesthai* to recall or remember. The Sanskrit word *manas* means *mind* or *sense*. The Indo-European word *minden* means to *remember, remind, notice*, or *turn one's attention to*. A *mind* is also defined as: *that with which a person thinks; the incorporeal (nonmaterial) subject of the psychical faculties; mental or psychical; to attend to, give heed to; being;* and *to perceive, to have one's attention caught by*.

We can draw on several of these definitions. *Memory* – the mind is connected to the past. *Thinking* – the mind becomes the tool of thought (the antithesis of *emptiness*). The words *think* and *remember* have the same root. Thought therefore is based on past experience and cannot be relied upon for self-transcendence. To *notice* or *turn one's attention to* is more positive. The mind cannot directly transcend itself, because its contents are the result of past experiences and expectations based on those experiences. But the mind can notice itself within consciousness and can be attentive to itself by directing consciousness. Change occurs in the act of noticing.

The mind and consciousness may attend to each other, but consciousness is the underlying predominant force.

DIVIDING THE INDIVISIBLE

Yogis attempted to transcend the mind and dynamize consciousness. The attentive mind can enter its conditioned aspects to reveal pure consciousness. Consciousness can then deliver a deeply present way of being that disperses all superfluous activity. Consciousness does the work.

Brains and minds

I cannot feel my brain but am aware of my mind and consciousness. However hard I think, I cannot feel my brain thinking. When teaching I am unaware of a brain. I know it is there but I cannot feel it. However deeply we go, I cannot feel the tissues of my brain as I can my skin or breath. Being unable to feel my brain in no way affects the quality of the work. Laing's *The Divided Self* makes no reference to brain parts or chemistry, but directs attention to the possibilities that arise when people are listened to. Krishnamurti and Rajneesh made no reference to the neurological circuitry of consciousness; it was not their job. Their fundamental interest lay in drawing attention to the potential changes that come from examining the subjective nature of experience. The study of the brain is necessary but beyond our sensory experience. Understanding brain anatomy and physiology does not change the quality of consciousness as we work. Our focus is the nature of experience through attention, a science in itself.

Antonio Damasio writes: "It is nice to know a little bit about how the brain does its job, but it is not necessary at all to experience anything. It will be even nicer to know more about the brain but not because that will be helpful at all to experience the world" (Damasio 2000).

Divisions of the mind are more relevant to our experience, although conclusions remain hypothetical. There have been no

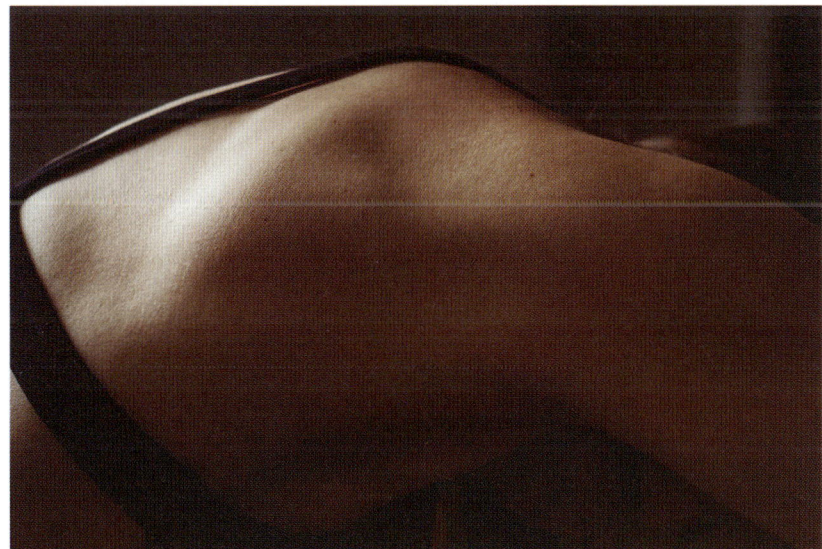

The attentive mind can enter its conditioned aspects to reveal pure consciousness. Consciousness can then deliver a deeply present way of being that disperses all superfluous activity. Consciousness does the work.

Chapter 4

major breakthroughs in understanding the mind since Freud wrote in 1940:

We know two things concerning what we call our psyche or mental life: firstly, its bodily organ and scene of action, the brain, (or nervous system), and secondly, our acts of consciousness, which are immediate data and cannot be more fully explained by any kind of description. Everything that lies between these two terminal points is unknown to us and, so far as we are aware, there is no direct relation between them. If it existed, it would at most afford an exact localization of the processes of consciousness and could give us no help toward understanding them. (Freud in Lowen 1958)

The depth mind

Freud suggested states and divisions of mind still in use today. He proposed that while some aspects of the unconscious were unavailable to awareness, others were available within a *preconscious* mind, implying that the subconscious and conscious were linked preconsciously. The preconscious mind held repressed material that could be released into consciousness to be assimilated and processed. He wrote: "The state in which ideas existed before being made conscious is called by us repression, and we assert that the force which instituted the repression and maintains it is perceived as resistance during the work of analysis. Thus we obtain our concept of the unconscious from the theory of repression" (Freud 1927/1962).

Repressed material reflects a conditioned state of not wanting to feel, not knowing how to feel, and not realizing that more might be felt. There are endless patterns of conditioning, imposed by belief systems, culture, ideas on living, and personal history that lie outside the scope of psychoanalysis. These include the mind's fundamental resistance to being and remaining quiet. The mind is distracted. Freud's theory of repression is relevant as experience deepens.

As we go inward, through the tissues, into the mind and consciousness, forgotten or repressed experiences come to light. Non-material realities surface as a consequence of involuntary physical expansion. Georg Feuerstein writes: "Long before modern psychology, Patanjali invented the significant concept of the 'depth mind,' which he called smriti (literally 'memory'). It is in the depth mind that the psychic residue of one's actions and experiences is stored" (Feuerstein 2003).

Jean Gebser was dismissive of psychology, writing: "much that sails under the name of psychology is a lesser but nevertheless destructive demonology, for as long as phenomena remain unintelligible and unrecognized, their effect on us will be disruptive" (Gebser 1949/1985).

But Feuerstein points out that: "The depth mind is not simply a bottomless ditch into which the content of our self-expression is dumped. But is an active force, the nurturing ground that engenders new impulses towards self-expression" (Feuerstein 2003). He highlights the emergence of an insightfulness freed from the constraints of conditioned patterning. The depth mind is active. Insight bubbles up from beneath the surface. People experience flashbacks, relive past events, and may have feelings of shame, fear, anger, or loss, often followed by a sense of deep self-forgiving, an aspect of emotional and spiritual healing.

Dividing the indivisible

The depth mind resonates with Freud's preconscious and subconscious mind. Freud used an intellectual approach to understand psychoemotional pathology. His psychoanalytical technique was based on his understanding of depth psychology. Yoga, on the other hand, has had little interest in content. It has been more concerned with freeing us from repetitive conditioned activity, regardless of its source.

Selves

Consciousness and the mind enable a sense of self. A self is deeply rooted in consciousness but is not all of consciousness. *Sense of self* is imperative, otherwise we would just be consciousness, which is the yoga ideal and a place worth visiting, if only to say we have been there. There appears to be a variety of selves interwoven within consciousness.

The Shorter Oxford English Dictionary defines a self as:

- "That which in a person is really and intrinsically he."

- "A permanent subject of successive and varying states of consciousness," implying that our selves are subjected to consciousness. This may be so, but the self also imposes upon the deeper qualities of consciousness.

- "An assemblage of characteristics and dispositions which may be conceived as constituting one of various conflicting personalities within a human being," acknowledging that things are far from simple.

A self is personal to its owner, we *have* a self. A self is the center of its own experience and subject to the pull of feelings and circumstances. We operate from a sense of self. Developmental psychologists suggest that we have developed a self by the time we are 18 months old, and perhaps even earlier. We *develop* a self. Selves are not implicit at birth (Kagan in Damasio 2000). The yoga experiment initially requires a clear, undiluted sense of self in order to accept the unaccustomed freedom that arises in tandem with spatial and dynamic consciousness.

Selfhood is a term used to denote having a self. The word *hood* from the Old English *hode* means *protection*, suggesting that *selfhood* is external, protective of something beneath it, an adornment hiding our truer selves. Selves may not run smoothly. Our sense of self relies on an identity resulting from and feeding a conditioned idea of who we are in our own eyes and who we appear to be in the eyes of others. Identity is essential and reinforced by achievements, work, interests, possessions, the confirmation of others, and relationships. We are aware of our identity, but often unaware of the extent of its conditioning. A deeper sense of self loosens a need to prop up our identity. We can transcend identification without abandoning our individuality. We can celebrate our identity without resorting to overidentification.

Various selves occupy individual consciousness and may follow us into practice. We might penetrate several selves as consciousness intensifies. What kinds of selves constitute a total sense of self? How many selves are we aware of as experience deepens? Some may be more obvious than others.

Chapter 4

When we cut through it all it may not matter. It is interesting to note the nature of selves that contribute to our conditioned and unconditioned experience.

We work with groups of selves. Groups experience the self of the teacher. There is much more beneath the surface of a self.

False and true selves

The false self is a camouflage, disguising, if and when necessary, our true feelings, opinions, and observations. We are aware of the convenience afforded by a false self. The false self is a consequence of socialization, expediency, politeness, the necessity to be less than honest, and wanting others to think well of us. The false self is built on the quality of the true self.

True selves represent an inner behavior not revealed to others. We are (usually) aware of our true self and its ambiguity, but may be less aware of the extent of its conditioning. True selves are opposed to our *true nature* which is unconditioned. A schism can develop between the true and false selves over "what people think." Someone revealing all the content of her true self might find the world a lonely place.

Laing observed that "dividing the self" was a defensive maneuver aimed at preserving the true self while offering to the world an ambassador: the "false self." "Accordingly this painful process involves a split in a mind and a body, an identification with the mind and a split from the body" (Clay 1996).

The true self censors external behavior as we slip between what we do and do not show. Conditioning may be so well established in some people, they believe their false self in part to be their true self.

Calming, softening, and opening together surrenders the false self, allowing the positive aspects of the true self to emerge. Ambiguities dissolve as altruistic feelings come to the foreground.

Large and small selves

We are familiar with the large and small selves that conceptualize yoga, and can observe and refer to the ongoing exchange between them. The small self is the habituated, familiar self, while the large self implies an enlightened altruistic self with an invested interest in a universal picture. The large self engages a transcendent experience as a part of a perceived cosmic reality. The large self penetrates the conditioning imposed by the small, false, and true selves to reveal an uncluttered self with spiritual confidence. The larger self that we notice ourselves *becoming* is not separated from its immediate or worldly environment.

We are not asking students to discover something they may be unaware of, but simply drawing attention to their inner witness, implicit since childhood, and suggesting they may use it coherently as a means for promoting a more enlightening experience. Dissolving impeding selves requires noticing and

DIVIDING THE INDIVISIBLE

passing through reactions and responses as they arise.

> When lucid, calmly distinguish between your false and true, small and large selves.

Deeper selves and consciousness

The true, false, and small selves eclipse a pre-existent deeper self that emerges in fits and starts before sustaining itself for longer periods. Passing through tissue sensation takes us into, and through, superficial selves. Penetrating materiality penetrates nonmateriality. As the mind empties it awakens to deeper tissue sensations, and the sensations in turn deepen consciousness. Analysis and content are replaced by lucid space as the mind rests quietly within consciousness and within the body.

Consciousness is phased, each phase having evolved out of and still containing its precedent. The self as we know it has developed out of these phases. A deeper self is bathed in the less sullied original phases of consciousness. Neuroscientist Antonio Damasio suggests that each developing phase of consciousness consolidates the evolution of a new self which forms a basis for the next evolving phase of consciousness, which in turn leads to the further development of a more evolved self, and so on.

Selves and consciousness have enabled each other. Both have relied on sensory input from the body. Damasio acknowledges that *attention* has been fundamental to this process. Consciousness and selves developed from attention to *something*. Our work uses sensation and mental content as objects of attention.

By *dropping down* into and beyond deeper sensations we reach a unified feeling, a *knowing* relationship, between the superficial selves and those buried by conditioning. Because we are conscious of *being* a self, consciousness and selfhood can be separated in awareness, we can observe how they feed each other. Attention to sensation and consciousness penetrates conditioning and draws us into deeper realms of experience. We can use the deeper extent of the self to penetrate and dissolve conditioned responses.

Other selves

Antonio Damasio proposes that there are other selves that correspond to parallel phases of consciousness. Some are available to conscious awareness and some are not. Three of these selves are described below.

Protoself

A protoself lies beneath conscious awareness, is unconditioned, and made up of neural patterns representing the state of the organism. The protoself is deeply enfolded within consciousness, has no powers of perception, and has no knowledge but may provide a primitive sense of self through sensation. It has been an essential factor in the development of consciousness.

Core self

A core self may be available to conscious awareness and is stimulated and generated

Chapter 4

by an object, and is continuous in time. We might experience core consciousness as an awareness of being in time with time as we follow sensation. A core self resonates with Jean Gebser's magical consciousness. It feels as if the mind touches a core self as it enters the deeper reaches of consciousness.

Autobiographical self

An autobiographical self is available to conscious awareness, is based on core self-experiences, and can be modified by further experience. The autobiographical self involves well-established behavior, has memory, and can anticipate the future. It holds personal history, grows with life experience, and can be conditioned but can also change to accommodate new experiences. An autobiographical self is synonymous with integral consciousness.

Interrelated phases of consciousness and selves appear to be loosely organized in layers or enfoldments reflecting their evolutionary hierarchy. They arise from one another, remain intimately continuous, and relate to the body sensations that contribute to our sense of self. We knowingly or unknowingly pass through these phases. The unification of all phases of consciousness and selves culminate in a private self which has a universal experience. The flow between them and their combined influence may manifest as light bulb moments, insights, or the more sustained experience of realization and *knowing*.

We consciously or unconsciously connect with deeper aspects of consciousness.

It is unclear which aspects may come to awareness, hence the suggestion that there is only one consciousness. We might drop into an intensely private space, free from all considerations – a so-called universal experience.

We might acknowledge phases of consciousness and interactive selves and mull over *how we happen to be as we are*. Enhancing spatial consciousness may be enough to get on with. Immediate experience can show a sensory, emotional, and intellectual self. We can tune into an attentive, quiet self, and may notice a vulnerable or visionary self. We might move between a playful, doubtful, anxious, excited self or observe a suspicious, expectant, impatient, creative, or loving self, *all in passing*. We may arrive at a self that is devoid of what we think of as our self.

I am

The ego is cited as the major impediment to progress. If Freud had not suggested an ego, we might not know that we had one, but we would know that we had our selves. *Ego* the Latin for *I am* or *the I*, was a term coined by Freud in the 1920s to denote our conscious experience of ourselves and ourselves in relation to the world. He acknowledged the ego as the essence of mental life. For Freud the ego represented the upper layer of consciousness experiencing itself as being separated from other minds. Our egos test the reality of our experience. In this respect, experience needs to be authentic. The developing ego has been the essential aspect of our progress, but due to its nature it also inhibits progress.

Dividing the Indivisible

The term ego implies a separation from everything that lies beneath it. To an extent, it is separated. Separating an ego from the preconscious consciousness and unconscious enabled Freud to analyze material arising from beneath ego consciousness, but he was aware of the inseparability of the ego and the deeper layers of consciousness. For him, the division was a tool for analysis, but he was also aware of the problems of ego dominance. The idea of a separative ego is useful as it confirms our ability to look at our behavior.

Freud observed: "In the course of our development we have effected a separation of our mental existence into a coherent ego and into an unconscious and repressed portion which is left outside it; and we know that the stability of this new acquisition is exposed to constant shocks" (Freud 1927/1962). Freud's observation implies that in consolidating itself the ego has rendered itself fragile, susceptible to the swings of life and to the consequences and awareness of our feelings. We have bitten the apple from the tree of knowledge.

Looking inward, we notice a behaviorist and its witness. Our witness observes our feelings, mental activity, actions, reactions, and responses. For most of us this has been clear since childhood. We are usually aware of how we are and how we behave.

The ego has many functions and duties, of which noticing our inner life is one of the most essential. Noticing gives the opportunity to enhance the quality of relationships with ourselves and with others and forms the basis for esoteric traditions and practices. When consciousness observes its ego, the intelligence of the ego observes itself. As Alexander Lowen put it: "the ego is a perception of perception, a consciousness of consciousness" (Lowen 1958). The tool we use to acknowledge the ego is the ego itself. The term ego is used as a synonym for the self in the subjective sense. "Here again, the difficulty in knowing the self through the self is apparent. Yet this is the only way, for the ego is the first thing we encounter as we turn inward on ourselves" (Lowen 1958).

The term *ego* can give a false impression of an entity set apart from the foundations and scope of consciousness. Ego denotes activities that occur within the upper reaches of consciousness but remains a consequence of our evolution and is inseparable from the deeper reaches of consciousness. Like the branch of a tree, the ego is continuous with its deep roots, arising from an archaic consciousness, a protoself, and culminating in a full-blown self. The roots are intact and present but superseded by more recent characteristics that hover between subconscious origins and our potential for dynamic consciousness.

The ego has as its nucleus the system of perception and embraces the conscious, but this should be extended to include all that was once conscious - the repressed unconscious and the preconscious. (Freud 1927/1962).

The ego is the greatest achievement of consciousness, the pinnacle of the latter's evolutionary journey, but it has characteristics that are the antithesis of everything yoga

Chapter 4

aspires to. Classical yoga and psychoanalysis accepted the ego's essentiality for human progress while acknowledging certain aspects as obstructive to personal development. The essential tool of consciousness, as with any tool, is subject to misuse.

The ego is the agent of the individual, the great divider, separating us from one another. Yoga scholar Georg Feuerstein writes: "In effect, the ego is a process. It is our activity of differentiating ourselves from 'other' beings and things. It is the way in which we choose, in every moment, to relate to the world as separate identities" (Feuerstein 1997).

It is not surprising that yoga sees the ego as a device apt to lose its way and favors its transcendence. We are never completely egoless. We may transcend rational consciousness to a point but the ego remains in the background recording the experience. Moderate transcendence softens the ego's grip, teaching us how to use it wisely. The ego is not only needed for navigating life but also in practices that temper the ego itself. The ego in refined form is the gateway to spatial and dynamic consciousness.

Lowen wrote:

the ego is more than the light in the darkness of the unconscious ... it controls motility ... Within limits, the ego can release an action or hold it back until conditions are opportune. It can inhibit actions and even repress them beyond consciousness ... The ego is like a light which is turned both outward and inward. Outwardly it searches the environment through the senses; inwardly it comprises a set of signals which govern outgoing impulses. (Lowen 1958)

The ego accepts or discards information from our external and internal world, monitoring how we feel and directing how we should proceed. It is our organizer, manager, discriminator, evaluator, and witness, enabling us to choose how to be from one moment to the next.

The ego decides how and when to connect with others, when to join group experience, and how to hold a group. A group is a collection of egos of differing intensities, varying histories, needs, and shades of experience.

> Go into the "I am" you know yourself to be. Can you recognize a condensation of activity representing you?

Freud cited the ego as the seat of anxiety. The seeds of anxiety have fertile soil. The development of the ego begins with contact with the mother's body and is bound up with fundamental anxieties around birth, *even when things go well*. Subsequent life experiences may be superimposed onto anxiety patterns from birth experience, stored in the unconscious, and, under given circumstances, arise into the ego for expression.

A strong ego is a sign of emotional health but we may have overencapsulated ourselves by developing a selfish and self-referential ego and, in the process, impeded an outgoing expansive self. A clear sense of ego centers around a healthy interaction with oneself

DIVIDING THE INDIVISIBLE

and others and is well equipped to manage the emotional shifts related to transformational experiences.

I am provides a reference point within consciousness. Practice reminds us of the ego's constant presence as it directs us, gets in our way, and as we use it to sift through what is wanted or unwanted. The ego can move fluidly between control, registration, adaption, acceptance, and surrender. As with stubborn or lazy tissue, the ego can be a door or a barrier to a deep experience. The ego decides to address itself by penetrating its own conditioned elements. During moments when we are immersed in spatial consciousness, the ego in modified form guides others and describes ongoing experience. Out of the ego comes Freud's "ego ideal," which is responsible for moral conscience, censorship, and negotiating unwanted instinctual needs or desires. Freud may have been unaware he was describing a code of behavior belonging to Eastern philosophy.

The ideal ego is quietly present, waiting to act if and when necessary. Our egos, along with rational consciousness, are to some extent fragmented. Once we discover that our self, our mind, and our ego are within consciousness it is clear that all three are fragmented. We only need look at the mind jumping from one thing to the next and back again, with little if any space around or between its contents, to realize that in general terms our minds are caught up in a zigzag of activity considered normal by most. Until it stops!

The ego must come together in some kind of unity before we can transcend it to some degree. An integrated ego, self, or mind responds more readily to the unfolding of the consciousness it inhabits. The first step is noticing and the second is calming things down in order to bring them into a workable unity.

The ego and sensation

Ego development is stimulated following birth, by skin-to-skin contact with the mother, producing a sense of *I am*. The surface of the

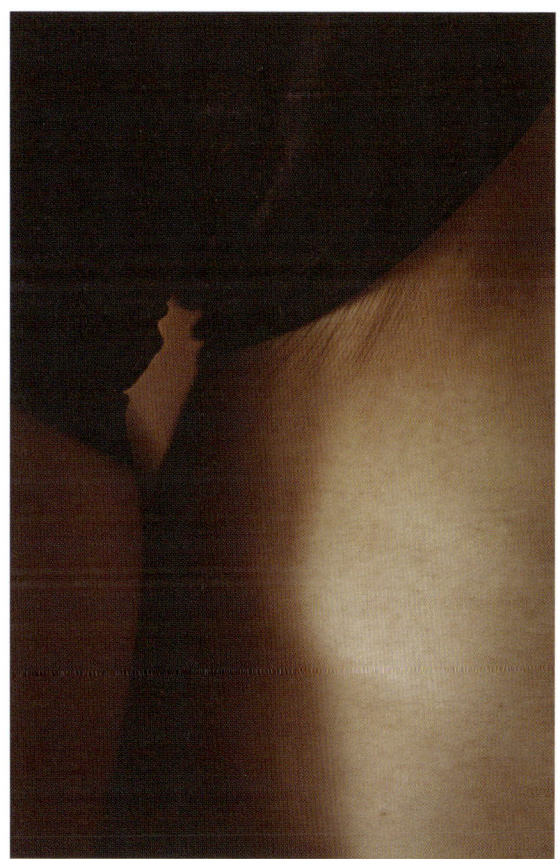

Skin expansion and ego expansion are involuntary movements that affect each other. The ego follows the skin.

Chapter 4

body is a reservoir of sensory patterning connecting to inner life. Alexander Lowen concurred with Freud that:

the ego is derived from body sensation, springing chiefly from the surface of the body ... Experiments have confirmed the fact that sensation occurs when an internal movement reaches the surface of the body and of the mind where the system perception conscious is located ... We can through the body dig down deeply into the less conscious aspects of ego supremacy and invite unconditioned elements of being to surface. (Lowen 1958)

Mysticism acknowledges a constantly changing body unable to sustain a fixed identity. Iyengar wrote: "Early yoga philosophers identified a grey area between what is me and not me, something that can be either or both, an interface between 'I'-ness and the outer world. It is my body. The great attention that yoga, and other practices too, pay to the body derives from its paradoxical position" (Iyengar 2005).

Freud wrote:

A person's own body, and above all its surface, is a place from which both external and internal perceptions may spring. It is seen like any other object, but to the touch it yields two kinds of sensations, one of which may be equivalent to an internal perception ... The ego is first and foremost a bodily ego; it is not merely a surface entity, but is itself the projection of a surface. ... not only what is the lowest but what is highest in the ego can be unconscious ... it is as if we were thus supplied with a proof of what we have just asserted of the conscious ego; that it is first and foremost a body-ego. (Freud 1927/1962)

There is a soft line between sense of self and ego identity (self-reference). Sense of self is consolidated by blending physical sensation with the *feeling* of consciousness.

Ego identity is loosened as we pass through tissue engagement. Tissue sense provides an anchor from which the ego can recede, enabling consciousness to expand and deepen.

> Move your awareness inward through the surface of your body. Blend the physical sensations with sensations of consciousness. Feel a heightened sense of self spread through your tissues and out into your immediate environment. Notice a deeper sense of self.

The ego and expansion

The ego can be contractive or expansive. Defensive patterns, excessive self-reference, and anxiety are *contractive*, while self-realization, yielding, and insightfulness are *expansive*. Creative engagement invites an involuntary expansion to the body's surface. Involuntary expansion is the pleasurable expression of life.

The ego and skin mirror each other in expansion. Expansion of the skin draws the ego into expansion and loosens its grip. Feeling the skin as one continuous piece, melding areas of engagement with the skin

DIVIDING THE INDIVISIBLE

as a whole, diffuses the impeding aspects of the ego. Skin expansion and ego expansion are involuntary movements, each one affecting the other. The ego will follow its physical counterpart, the skin, and in turn the skin will expand in response to the diffusion of the ego. The ego follows the skin's sensory integration. It responds in kind. The mind learns from the sensations. Once the ego has unified, it can expand and enable spatial and dynamic consciousness to come through. Expansion is felt as an *indefinite* movement in all directions. The ego is drawn outward into an *infinite* expression as it follows an *indefinite* expansive movement of surface tissue.

When the ego expands it moves outward into the field of expansive consciousness. When threatened, the ego draws away from the broader field of expansive consciousness. We can feel the difference between expansive and contractive consciousness.

The ego and resistance

Tissue engagement may mirror the psycho-emotional resistance common to psychoanalysis. Initial resistance to expansion is an attempt to sustain the grip of identification. Gentle engagement at first stimulates the ego. The engagement must be appropriate for expansion to occur spontaneously.

As expansion takes over, spatial consciousness intensifies and identification weakens. We enter deeper consciousness and a profound sense of self engages with preconscious activity.

Our work converts engagement into expansion. Lowen observed: "The ego can release an action or hold it back until conditions are opportune. It can inhibit actions and even repress them beyond consciousness" (Lowen 1958). It is clear that excessive engagement represses action and that expansion is an action that releases material stored by and beneath ego consciousness. The degree of engagement necessary to stimulate involuntary expansion may differ between individuals.

As engagement becomes expansion, some engagement is maintained at the center of the sensation. A gentle dispersive hub of engagement has a stabilizing influence. The center of radiation acts as a station, from which we can travel through the space of consciousness.

"The origin of the ego and the origin of the sense of reality are but two aspects of one developmental step. This is inherent in the definition of the ego as that part of the mind which handles reality" (Fenichel in Lowen 1958). Our body ego underpins our sense of reality.

> Sessions usually begin with the upper ego in ascendance. Move into your lower ego by drawing on deeper physical sensation and spatial consciousness. Communicate with the group externally through your presence and internally through your process. The group unites in spatial consciousness.

Chapter 4

The obstructive and constructive ego

Our "I-ness" is an identifier. We need to identify with a certain particularity in order to maintain biological and mental integrity. All this is to the good, so how is it that the words ego and egoistic carry such negative connotations? (Iyengar 2005)

Iyengar's question is understandable, but he knew that the ego inhibits progress: "Much of yoga practice and ethic is concerned with cutting the ego down to size and removing the veil of unknowing that obscures its vision. ... when ego is quiescent, consciousness senses the reality of the soul, and the light of soul expresses itself through the translucent consciousness" (Iyengar 2005).

The ego we possess may possess us. The ego is a growing force and continues to reinforce itself into advanced years (Lowen 1958). Its plasticity invites conditioning but also the possibility of transformative experiences. The ego rediscovers its roots by passing through its *I am*. The ego's lens of perception penetrates itself.

There is no egoless state, simply grades of ego. The sublimity of Krishnamurti's ego-consciousness gave him a highly refined experience that he could enter without meditation or technique. He just *went there* while his worldly ego enabled him to teach and give talks. A stable ego was traditionally recommended for beginning yoga because it supports the vulnerability that can arise during the dissolution of conditioning. We need stability to transcend our familiar selves and enter a less known or unknown way of being. A balanced ego holds us quietly within our sense of self, so that we may venture into the space of insight and realization.

We cannot override the ego but can soften and lighten its presence as it moves between obstructive and constructive behavior. The ego (the I am) is in the practice with us, assessing resistance, noticing the mind, monitoring or

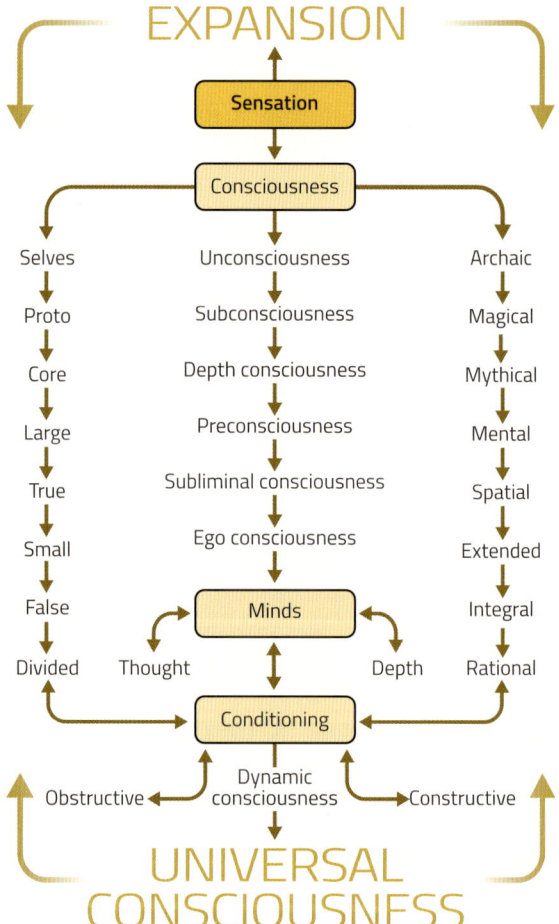

Categories of consciousness, minds, and selves.

DIVIDING THE INDIVISIBLE

congratulating itself on expansion. Its interference and its support vie for predominance. As we become less self-referential, the ego awakens to the preconscious and beyond.

> Soften your ego self as you enter inner space. Be inside and outside your body. Observe how your experience becomes less personal when tissues gently interface with your inner and outer space.

At worst the ego creates a contracted and separative existence; at best it expresses creative individuality while sustaining a unitive quality; beyond this, it acknowledges a field of consciousness, the origins of which remain a mystery.

Karma or conditioning

Patterns may be instilled by previous generations. Freud wrote:

The experiences of the ego seem at first to be lost for inheritance; but, when they have been repeated often enough and with sufficient strength in many individuals in successive generations, they transform themselves, so to say, into experiences of the id [Freud's term for the unconscious] the impressions of which are preserved by heredity. Thus in the id, which is capable of being inherited, are harboured residues of countless egos; … [the ego] may perhaps only be reviving shapes of former egos and be bringing them to resurrection. (Freud 1927/1962)

Freud's insight supports the "having been here before" or "where did that come from?" experience.

Georg Feuerstein, without reference to the ego but in accord with Freud, wrote:

Progress on the yogic path varies from person to person and depends on the individual's psychological capacity and, at a deeper level, his or her karma. Whatever we represent at the present moment is because of our past volitions … Our DNA is the product of the sum total of our karmic past, and so, according to Yoga, are our life circumstance and the experiences that we have and that impinge on us. Since much of what we call "mind" depends on brain functions and since our brain is DNA driven, our mental life too is largely determined by our karma. (Feuerstein 2003)

He goes on to acknowledge that our transcendent nature can overcome karmic baggage.

Top down, below up

Psychoanalysis is concerned with what is conscious and unconscious in mental life. Freud suggested that some elements of the unconscious were too deep to be made conscious, but that some could be made conscious because they could be accessed by the ego. He felt that much of the ego itself is unconscious and only a small part of it preconscious (Freud 1927/1962). Psychoanalysis starts from the top down, from upper egoic layers

55

Chapter 4

reaching down into subconscious or unconscious repressed activity in order to release it into awareness (for analysis). It is suggested that an unconscious and subconscious mind holds repressed material but that unconscious material is more deeply buried and more resistant to awakening. Yoga traditionally began from below up, by awakening the lower centers. Energy passing upward moved repressed activity into consciousness, giving little if any attention to its content.

Physicist Marilyn Ferguson quotes pioneering fellow physicist Karl Pribram: "Traditional theories of higher centers of the brain controlling lower ones was in need of radical modification. The older brain centers proved to have a richer complexity and more control than anyone had imagined" (Wilber 1982). This again resonates with Krishnamurti's experience that there is one consciousness.

The subconscious may also be conditioned. Bruce Lipton, author of *The Biology of Belief* (Lipton 2008), suggests that the subconscious holds a deeper conditioning. Old habits and beliefs about ourselves and the world are kept in the filing system of the unconscious. Subconscious material is pushed or drawn up as higher centers yield their inhibitions.

The ego acts as a tool and a teacher. Its roots run deeply down into the unconscious from where it sprang. An ego (us) extends downward and passes through older conditioned activity upon which our more recent conditioning may be based. Alexander Lowen wrote:

The ego must open up its barriers to allow experience in just as it must lower them to allow impulses out. The bigger the experience, the greater the experience must be. This is not a question of flexibility or adaptability, for these involve no change. Literally, an ego must allow itself to be overwhelmed by each new vital experience so that a new ego will arise in which that experience is properly integrated. But this is only possible when the ego extends in depth. (Lowen 1958)

Our experience reveals the fusion of an upward and downward movement as the older and more recent aspects of our conditioning pass through each other.

Consciousness and the body

The starting point for yoga's experiment is founded on a sense of self, confirmed by relationship to an object. Body sensation as the object provides a reflection in which consciousness can see itself. Physical engagement is an ideal object because it intensifies the reflection. We are our own mirror, engaging with sensation as the object of consciousness.

The degree to which the evolution of sensory tissue and the evolution of consciousness influenced each other is not known, but the correlation is undisputed. Incoming signals stimulated the awakening of what became a mind. In this respect the skin played a major role. Freud wrote: "An activity becomes conscious as it impinges on the surface of the body for only thus can it come into relation with the external world."

Lowen observed that the ego is a perceptual process and in civilized man is more than perception: "It is a perception of perception, a consciousness of consciousness, a self-consciousness" (Lowen 1958). Damasio also acknowledged consciousness as perception. Consciousness has evolved from perceptual sensation. As we tune in to, accept, and refer to heightened sensation we deepen the scope of consciousness. Consciousness evolved from living tissue, and its quality in turn changes living tissue. The relationship between our nonmaterial and material aspects *is the meditation*. We have one consciousness and one body with the dual plasticity for change. We can and do *dis*embody conditioning.

A welcome mystery

The unconscious is consciousness without awareness. In Freud's terms the unconscious and subconscious are aspects of consciousness devoid of awareness. Some might say we are partially unconscious and lack the awareness necessary for establishing more intelligent ways of being. Pure consciousness, empty in itself, drives us. Just beneath awareness lies an alternative state. Authorities divide consciousness but are unclear where the conscious ends and the subconscious begins (perhaps within the preconscious). So much *comes to mind* that has been enmeshed by memory and previous experience that it is impossible to say where the division lies. Reams of experience have been dispatched to the preconscious or unconscious. Who is to say what might surface, and how or when it may do so?

Philosopher William James favored the term *subliminal consciousness*. The Shorter Oxford English Dictionary defines the word *subliminal* as: "below the threshold of consciousness or sensation ... said of states to exist but not strong enough to be recognized." The word *sublime* is defined as "to raise to an elevated sphere or exalted state ... transmute into something higher, nobler or more excellent." These definitions suggest that subliminal consciousness lying just beneath awareness can reflect a purity or higher state. Subliminal consciousness also holds a reservoir of past experience. We dissolve the latter to highlight the former.

Consciousness is more expansive than the constructs that attempt to describe it. Dividing consciousness, minds, and selves is useful but pales in the light of direct experience. Consciousness gives space to *ideas* about consciousness, but the ideas become ever-receding objects. When we do not *seek* and are in the *present*, the *present* dissolves the conditioning containing the ideas. "The moment you give your total attention to your conditioning you will see that you are free from the past completely, that it falls away from you naturally" (Krishnamurti 1969).

I may well label group experiences as a mystic, magical, integral consciousness, or suggest an unconscious, sub, or preconscious, but I am also aware of an all-encompassing, deepening experience that includes wonder, amazement, the absence of thought, and a simultaneous blending with and separation from the group. When we have this alternative experience together, we may tune in to an ancient way of being, an archaic consciousness, or a core or protoself. But I have my self minus the clutter. I have my essential self as an aspect of unblemished consciousness.

Chapter 4

The reason for division is to put things back together with an understanding that may shed light on divergent behaviors we notice in ourselves and in others. Yoga masters, psychoanalysts, and quantum physicists divide consciousness in their own way. To a large extent they are saying the same thing, but their language and expressions differ.

It is not known how a mind experiences itself and experiences itself having experiences. Jean Gebser surmised: "Our own attempt at a synoptic view of the various consciousness structures, the various modes of existence and realization, has resulted in our construction of a 'synoptic table' precisely because these modes of existence and realization cannot be perceived systematically" (Gebser 1949/1985). In other words, divisions and phases of consciousness and selves are discretionary and cannot be pinned to a definitive conclusion.

Damasio states: "There is a mystery, however, regarding how images emerge as neural patterns … There is a gap between our knowledge of neural events, at molecular, cellular and system levels, on the one hand, and the mental image whose mechanisms of appearance we wish to understand" (Damasio 2000). There may come a time when this gap is found to contain an even more refined mix of neurobiological elements. Reducing the gap will not solve the mystery of human consciousness. The unknown is where we find the depth of the yoga experience.

Experiencing consciousness is like experiencing time, without breaks or interruptions, the present flowing from the past into the next moment. It feels like one fluid consciousness – a confluence of consciousnesses.

Profound realization occurs when attention to "how we are" is intensified. The relationship between sensation, consciousness, mind, and self is more fluid than their

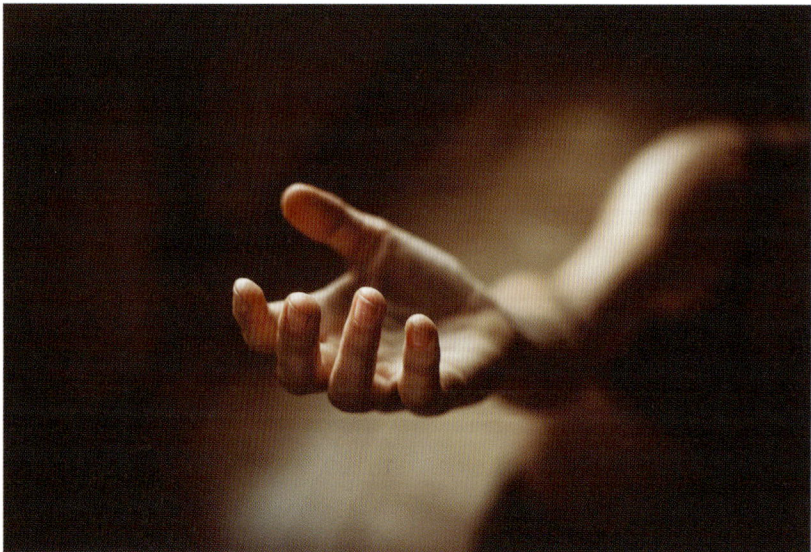

Profound realization occurs when attention to "how we are" is intensified. The relationship between sensation, consciousness, mind, and self is more fluid than their division implies.

Dividing the indivisible

division implies. As sensation varies in intensity, distribution, and scope so too does consciousness. Within a broad spectrum, it is all sensation and consciousness.

Unconditioned, uncluttered consciousness is an intensification coexistent with spatial expansion. Here is the starting point for understanding our experience, guiding others, and setting the stage for the arrival of insight and wisdom.

Dynamic consciousness

Dynamic consciousness is a shared experience highlighting the full potential of group presence. Dynamic consciousness is a surge, a swell, an outpouring of perceptual energy, a potency that pervades the cells, the entirety of experience, and the common space. Dynamic consciousness springs from the quiet unification of everything beneath, within, and around it and is the summit of the experience we return to time and again, a feature that sustains itself *when we remember its potential for doing so*. Dynamic consciousness arises from within spatial consciousness and is the pristine state of unconditioned awareness and attention. Perhaps all implicit phases of consciousness, minds, and selves contribute to dynamic consciousness through the direction of an ego free from thought. The ego initiates and receives dynamic consciousness, and could be overwhelmed were it not for an abiding sense of tissue and the density of surrounding space.

> A gentle inward shift of the mind, a decision made, unites sensation and spatial and dynamic consciousness. The experience sustains itself.

Manifest and nonmanifest

Manifest and nonmanifest are terms common to quantum physics and imply more subtlety than the terms material, or nonmaterial. They are useful in class work. The manifest encompasses everything known, all mental activity, and physical sensation. The nonmanifest is unknown, yet to be known, and unknowable. This kind of language is used by modern physics and mysticism. All things experienced or conjectured are manifest. Thought, consciousness, insight, and realization are manifest. Experience manifests out of unexperienced phenomena.

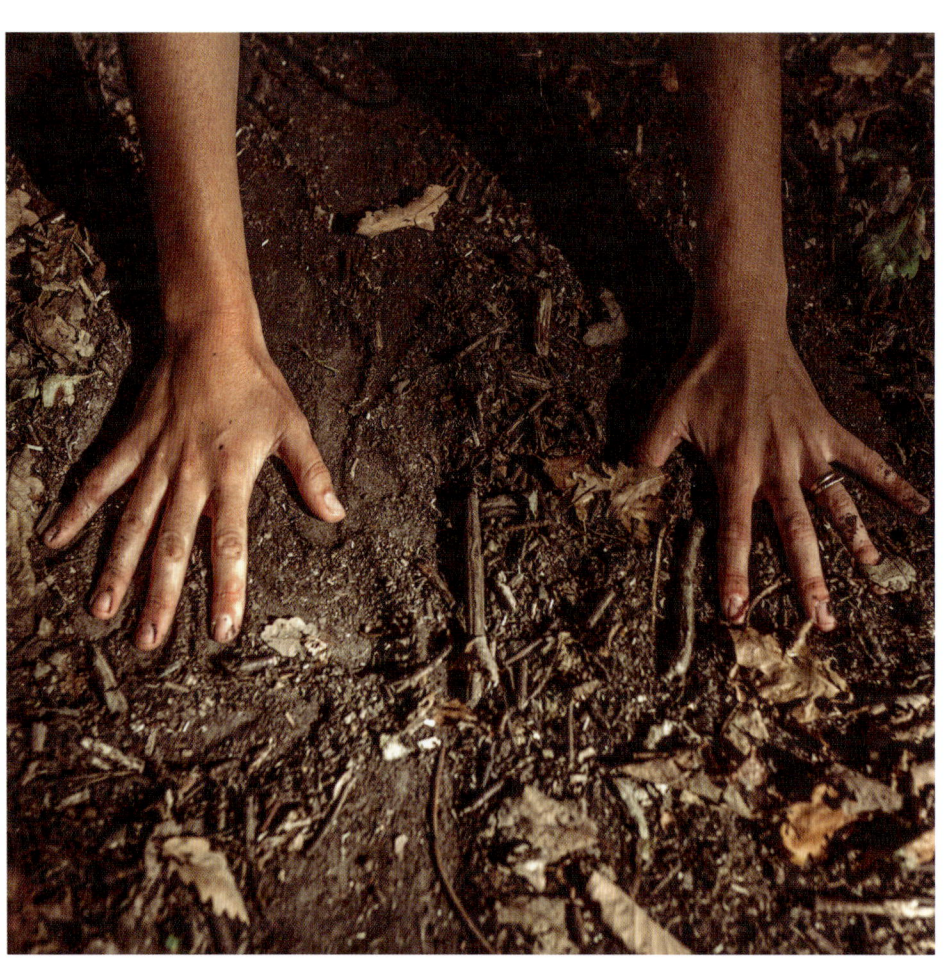

Sensing

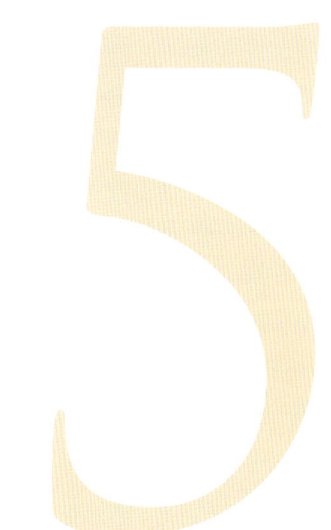

There are no courses, books, teachers, or methods that can transport us across the fine line between conditioned and unconditioned responses. Only we, quietly and unaided, can sense our way beyond the threshold into as yet undiscovered space.

A closer look

Maggie Gill is a craniosacral practitioner and teacher in the John Upledger tradition. We have a practitioner's dialogue. She asks questions while listening with her hands. Some years back during a session I asked her why she had followed through on something I had said. She said she had felt my tissues change as I recalled a specific event. I had not felt the changes nor was I aware the conversation was that significant. I was intrigued at the finer level of subtlety between mind and body.

The world is full of magic things, patiently waiting for our senses to grow sharper.

—W. B. Yeats

I began to look more closely. I was familiar with a deepening relationship between my mind and body but now fine-tuned my perception. Living tissue responds to the slightest thought, feeling, intimation, or anything seen as content within an empty mind. Mental activity, the slightest registration, related or unrelated to the work at hand, involves a parallel activity within the tissue, as if tissue thinks. Tissues are responsive to how we are from moment to moment, a material barometer of nonmaterial activity. There appears to be an unlimited potential for heightening body–mind sensitivity. There are advanced postures, breathing techniques, and meditations. There is also a spectrum of "advanced sensations" that come to light when called upon. Their awakening has a bearing on the quality of consciousness.

Sensing and sensation

There is a difference between sensing and sensation. We *do* sensing, it is an act, we sense our way into something, and we *receive* a sensation as a consequence. The sensation itself is passive – it is a feeling. Inner sensing highlights underlying, ever-changing densities of tissue. As we become more sensitive, we notice that the deeper and finer aspect of

Chapter 5

tissue has a labyrinthine quality. Tissues feel multisensorial, as we sense into an endlessly active and immediately responsive meshwork, a delicate, intricate maze of sensation. We have a sense of ever-changing spatiality, blending with a fine web of tissue, continuously reorganizing itself in response to its needs and our interest and attention.

Engaging tissues excessively creates a traction that gives a sense of *densification*. Being in the "right place" with the tissue stimulates the required expansive involuntary response. Sensing is a two-way phenomenon. We can enter into sensation with our attention and invite sensation into our attention. Consciousness receives sensation. Refining sensation requires going where the sensory nerve endings are abundant and accessible, particularly the skin. Once you have focused on where the body is in space – its position, shape, or range of movement – give your attention to surface activity, to how it informs and guides you. Surface sensation is primary. Other factors may be relevant but are secondary. The skin is the first point of contact with the ground. It moves with the breath and senses the space around it. It is important to remember that as we approach the tissues they are engaging and disengaging in countless ways before we start. It is easy to impose on this unpredictable activity, in the same way that it is easy to impose a meditation technique on a mind that is constantly changing tack, balancing, and rebalancing itself.

The relationship between our material and nonmaterial selves is optimized when we feel more. Sense of self arises from the relationship between consciousness and sensory awareness giving us the scope for deepening sensitivity on all levels. Awakening the body awakens consciousness and us.

Engage gently and quietly with your tissues. Allow them to inform you. Follow the relationship between consciousness and sensation. Take others into the experience with you.

Tissue and consciousness

We can give sensation precedence because sensation preceded consciousness in our development. We can use sensation to gain re-entry into the expansive depth of consciousness. Consciousness can then look at itself and sensation simultaneously. The art is to settle on sensation without thought. Tissue changes texture of its own accord as we observe its behavior. Tissue knows how to respond to uncluttered focused consciousness.

Consciousness is a sensation we can feel. The feeling of consciousness merges with the sense of tissue expansion as one spatial dimension, one sensation. Antonio Damasio writes:

In the end consciousness begins as a feeling, if it feels like a feeling it may well be a feeling … By making feelings be the primitives of consciousness we are obliged to inquire about the intimate nature of feeling. (Damasio 2000)

Sensing

Mysticism and modern physics suggest that matter is and is of consciousness, implying that tissue *may have consciousness* and be *part* of a grand consciousness, in the same way that a tree, cloud, or lake might have consciousness. The difference being that living human tissue is closer to personal consciousness. The physicist David Bohm commented:

the more complex an animal the greater its display of intelligence, but the intelligence must also be immanent in the matter that constitutes the animal. If the immanence is pursued more and more deeply in matter, I believe we may eventually reach the stream which we also experience as mind, so that mind and matter fuse. (Bohm and Weber in Wilber 1982)

Background activity

As we proceed it is clear that consciousness is awash with background activity. Shadowy thoughts, half thoughts, intimations, and emotions dance with background sensations that include rhythms, pulsations, waves, and miscellaneous self-regulatory activities. A refined study discovers an ever-changing fusion of mental, emotional, and physiological activity. The philosopher William James recognized that feelings are a reflection of body state changes. The balance between tissue sensation and how we feel continually shifts. Background feelings and mental activity are always present to give us the *feeling of being present*. We do not have to act on the activity but by going into sensations and the mind simultaneously, we dissolve the experience, we transcend ourselves.

> Go into a position you can spend a little time in. What do you notice as you settle and sensation comes to the foreground? Perhaps a myriad of background activity, eddies, pulsations, and waves that defy definitive description. Become aware of the finer mental and emotional activity that is corresponding to subtle changes in the tissue. We are sentient beings drawing on our capacity for finer and finer sensation.

Primary and secondary sensation

Applying gentle engagement brings primary sensations to the foreground of awareness. Areas of primary sensation invite secondary sensation throughout neighboring areas and throughout the body as a whole. Secondary sensations accompany primary sensations, indicating an awakening sensory system. Tissue over the thighs may produce primary sensations while shoulder tissue may produce secondary sensations, and vice versa. As creative engagement disperses, secondary sensations move to the foreground of awareness, revealing the potential for a practice that moves between primary and secondary sensations. At some point the entire body takes part in the action. Follow the sensations, go where they take you. Interest and attention facilitate involuntary activity.

Experiencing tissue

Sensation and consciousness touch. The sensory mind by definition is more sensitive than the thinking mind. Thinking about

Chapter 5

sensation enhances it, but will inhibit it at some point. Applying sensory thought to an area is productive to a degree (softening the belly, widening the back of the waist). Once the sensation is up and running sensory thought loses its effect and impedes progress. Sensation should take over from sensory thought for the process to sustain itself. Sensation free from sensory thought opens consciousness.

The mind might not do the job to begin with (but can). We can soften initial resistance or recurrent stiffness with a few breaths. But once the tissues have opened, the additional sensation of the breath can distract from the fine exclusive focus needed for the tissues. We can't go slowly enough. Going slowly, almost too slowly for the conditioned mind tempers the ego. The sense of *I am* is a body sense as we engage the tissues. Engaging the skin as one continuous piece unifies the fragmentation of the ego. The ego can only release its grip when it feels totally unified with the body.

Sentience

Normal consciousness implies we are awake, alert, have our wits about us, and can think and make decisions. Consciousness enables self-awareness and creativity (creative self-awareness). *Sentience* is defined as *the capacity to feel, perceive, or experience subjectively:* a definition that recognizes our creative potential for inspired teaching. An Eastern definition of *sentience* describes *a metaphysical quality of all things deserving respect.*

Sensory physiology within tissues does not *appear* to be consciously aware of its own perceptivity. Living tissue has contributed to the development of consciousness but in itself is not endowed with consciousness as we know it. Tissue cannot think, rationalize, or make decisions, but tissue can *feel* sentient to practitioners with advanced levels of

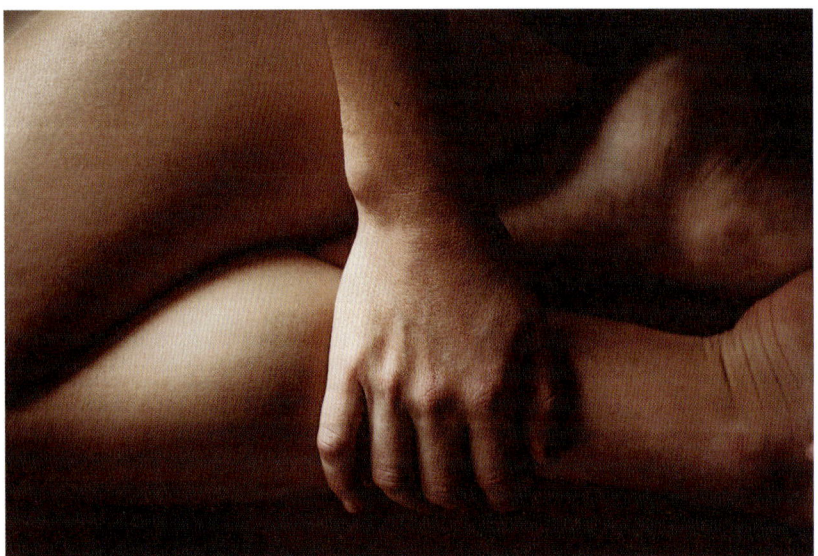

Engaging and sensing the skin as one continuous piece unifies the fragmentation of the ego.

SENSING

sensitivity. Tissue's responsiveness and sensitive presence gives it sentient possibilities, as if it subjectively feels and might be aware of itself feeling, or sense us sensing it.

Consciousness can enter the body so completely we get the impression that tissue is sentient – a feeling that grows the more we stand back and subjectively observe tissue's behavior. Conscious awareness and sensation feel as one. The more attention we give to tissue the more we suspect its sentience. Consciousness itself can be perceived as a sensation.

The sensory mind–brain and thinking mind–brain differ functionally but belong to the same mind–brain. They blend and cross-refer, informing each other on a continual basis. Some areas predominantly think, some predominantly feel, while some areas think and feel. We can feel without thinking but cannot think without feeling. All thought has a sensory component. The body feels our thoughts. When thought is absent feeling is present in some form or another. Pathology or trauma aside, consciousness and sentience are inseparable. We are sentient beings endowed with consciousness. Sentience is a primitive form of consciousness. During the finer moments of practice, it feels as if tissue has consciousness. Over and above our imagination, the following point to this possibility:

- Consciousness has evolved from sensory input from the body.

- Sensory activity within and beneath awareness is a primitive form of consciousness.

- Sensation comes *into* consciousness.

- Brain tissue and body tissue are neurologically and biochemically linked.

- Membranous, fascial, and extremely fine connective tissue is continuous between and throughout the brain and the body, from the skin to the deepest areas of the brain and back again.

- The mind is fed by a brain composed of neural tissue intimately tied to neuromuscular, neurofascial, and neurodermal tissue, all having evolved from one neurogenic fabric. We have only one nervous system regardless of its origins and categorizations.

- Tissues respond to the *content* of thought. Thinking soft or light, softens and lightens the tissues. As they soften and lighten, so does consciousness.

- The delicately felt presence of tissue responsiveness suggests that tissue and consciousness are extensions of each other.

- Consciousness and tissue are nonmaterial and material reflections of each other.

- Consciousness can be perceived as a sensation. We feel conscious and feel consciousness.

Chapter 5

Antonio Damasio suggests that *how* consciousness emerges cannot be entirely answered by postulating a mechanism to wake up and energize the cerebral cortex, even though the cortex shows patterns of electrophysiological activity in the waking state. In his opinion this does not address the issue of self and *knowing* which he considers to be at the heart of consciousness. He suggests that consciousness arises from signals delivered to the brain (in order for it to regulate homeostasis) from the organism moment by moment (Damasio 2000).

The fact that consciousness arises from the body does not answer the question "is tissue conscious?" but comes close because consciousness can exist without thought or content to keep it going. Mental activity impedes the extraordinary sensitivity of living tissue. The more we dissolve mental content the more it seems that tissue has sentience. The more we awaken *a possibility* of tissue sentience, the more we dynamize consciousness. Tissue may not be consciously aware of itself, but its texture continuously and creatively responds to organic and mechanical needs and is responsive to, and provokes, emotional activity, background feelings, and thought. Tissue is sensitive to mental concentration, relaxation, analysis, and suggestion, giving the impression that tissue is conscious in some way. Living tissue expresses life and reflects consciousness. We *are* living tissue and consciousness. The idea, factual or not, that tissue in some way has consciousness, inspires us to listen to its subtle messages, and give it the respect it deserves.

Given the benefit of the doubt, tissue sensitivity and its direct link to the mind has a powerful effect on consciousness. Tissue sensation is at the other end of consciousness, and may have consciousness.

Tissue knows

Consciousness has a twofold aspect. There is first the consciousness of feelings and actions, and secondarily, the consciousness of knowing. (Lowen 1958)

As we heighten sensitivity it feels as if tissue knows us, and the vital presence of tissue enhances the feeling of *knowing*. All aspects of ourselves are put in perspective by a spectral sense of *knowing* submerged beneath a tide of rational consciousness. Sensation and consciousness *know* each another. There is a crossover between *knowing* feeling, and feeling that we *know*. *Knowing* ourselves begins with the feeling of *knowing*, minus the content that clouds self-perception. Tissue may have a primitive sense of *knowing*, revealed by its tendency to *let us in*. Tissue reveals a sense of *knowing* that predates consciousness. Feeling is a way of knowing and *knowing* is consciousness.

This may be where the possibility of tissue consciousness exists. There is the potential that tissue is not only responsive to the mind but during its most sensitive state *knows* us. It detects our intention and sees us coming. If we accept uncluttered consciousness as "a sense of knowing," might there be a sense of knowing in the tissues? In the profundity of our most subtle moments, as density disperses, tissue *feels* as if it *knows*. If tissue, as an object of

Sensing

consciousness, has reflected consciousness back to itself, tissue may be conscious by default. Tissue does not have the sophisticated neural patterning of the brain but has played an integral part in its evolution, and continues to support our inquiry into alternative ways of being. Sensing the delicate interaction between mind and tissue gives the impression that tissues *know*. *Knowing* is consciousness.

At times it feels as if tissue knows more than the mind (a clumsy mind entering sensitive tissue). Tissue feels attentive, as if it listens to the mind. The deeper and more lucid our attention, the more we discover that tissue knows how to respond. We should proceed as if our tissues know us.

Sensation and emotion

Candace Pert writes: "The body is the unconscious mind! Repressed trauma caused by overwhelming emotion can be stored in a body part, thereafter affecting our ability to feel that part or even move it" (Pert 1998).

Emotions are sensations, and sensation has emotional content. When quietly deep, (or deeply quiet) we can sense our tissues reflect an ongoing tide of background emotion. Emotions were well established before the advent of conscious awareness. We become aware of feeling emotion as consciousness develops. Primary emotions such as fear, anger, love, joy, and sadness are usually (but not always) obvious. When the primary emotions are in abeyance, we might notice subtle emotional content. Expansion draws out background emotion. We might detect agitation, restlessness, dissatisfaction, hesitation, anticipation, disappointment, doubt, pride, avoidance, or slivers of understated excitement. Emotional content is ever present. As sensation becomes more pleasurable, positive background emotions replace those interfering with expansion.

In our usual everyday consciousness, we are not aware of the operations that produce the forms, transformations, and differentiations wherewith we perceive, think and feel, but we need not be, in an additional sense, cut off from them. (Laing 1982)

Background emotion is physically expressed by subtle musculoskeletal changes detected during periods of refined silence and attention. Thought induces a flow of background emotion underscoring internal behavior. Background emotion and thought are fundamental aspects of rational consciousness. They are potentially disruptive but are tempered and put in perspective by spatial consciousness. When tissues are expansive, soft, and light, we *feel* wise, calm, and *emote* insight and wisdom.

When we are "noticing" we discover that all experience has a subtle emotional substrate. Noticing subtle emotion indicates that deeper layers of conditioning are surfacing and dissolving. It is a process we go through time and again.

Chapter 5

> Engage your tissues while observing your state of mind. Be aware of the activity, related and unrelated to current sensations. Go into everything you notice without analysis. Pass through all background activity with clear attention. Feel your tissues change as mental activity and emotions disperse.

Sensory distinctions

We can sense tissue without having to refer to its physiology. We may be aware that some tissues are richly endowed with sensory nerve endings, that skin has more sensory nerve endings than muscle, and is the most readily accessible *feeler*. The scope of sensation is best understood subjectively by its effect on us and our effect on it. Sensitivity is reduced by an overload of tension but if underloaded lacks the stimulation it requires for transformative possibilities. Tissue sensitivity is enhanced by an approach acknowledging its sensitivity.

The skin is the most primitive sensory organ. The surface of the body responds to mental suggestion due to its rich nerve supply, its unbroken spread, and its embryonic unfoldment from the deep tissue comprising the central nervous system. The lightest touch from another person can light up the entire nervous system. Sensory tissue awakens the sensory mind, in turn awakening consciousness. Every surface sensory nerve passing through the central nervous system plays its part.

Many teachers have studied fascia and its role in sensory distribution. Fascial tissue, investing and carrying sensory nerves, weaves its way throughout the body in webs, strings, sheaths, bags, and cylinders, and on a finer level passes back into its deep central origin. This explains why persistent focus on the surface brings to awareness the shapes and movements of the deeper structures.

The most interesting research comes from French surgeon Jean-Claude Guimberteau. In the fascinating book, *Architecture of Human Living Fascia*, he confirms a feeling we have during our finer moments, one of total "tissular continuity." In effect, there is no surface tissue: the outer body is a continuous expression of tissue at all depths and densities. Guimberteau highlights structural and sensory continuity of surface tissues into the deepest centers of the body:

What impresses us most in this world of great mobility is the general suppleness of the epidermis and the dermis which can be folded and manipulated. There is no stratification and no separation between them. The movement of the dermis is continuous with the movements of the epidermis and hypodermis within this interwoven maze. Nerves are incorporated everywhere within this structure. (Guimberteau & Armstrong 2015)

He points out that the fine connective tissue network and its associated nerves are continuous, from the surface through the gross fascial structures, muscle, and into the underlying bone. The entire arrangement contributes to a sense of self and to an awakening consciousness.

SENSING

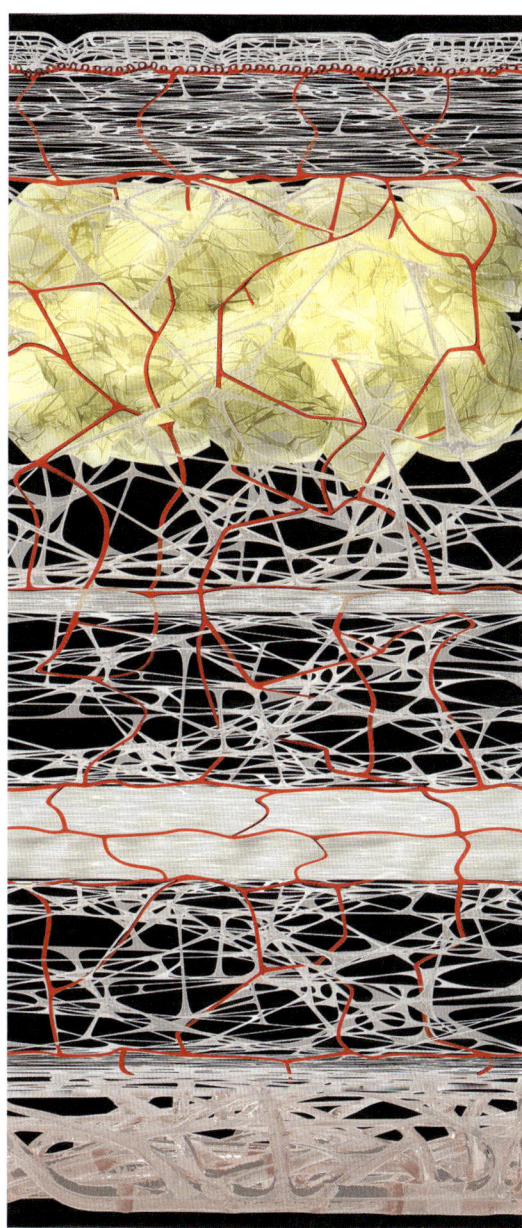

Epidermis to cancellous bone, showing the indivisibility and continuity between the fine surface and deep bone tissue (Guimberteau & Armstrong 2015).

Involuntary expansion

Involuntary activity played a significant role in the evolution of consciousness, as sensory signals stimulated our primitive organism. Tuning in to involuntary expression brings us closer to the origins of conscious awareness. Varying qualities of involuntary activity reveal themselves, and are magnified by clear and unwavering attention. Undisturbed focus on tissue *presence* reveals a proliferation of involuntary activity.

Consciousness itself is an involuntary phenomenon. We do not *decide* to become conscious any more than we decide to produce a cerebrospinal rhythm. The feeling of involuntary tissue expansion correlates with the transcendent yoga experience. We find ourselves *in expansion*. We cannot *do* expansion but can follow it. It is not stretching but may initially feel like the lightest stretch until we refine sensitivity. The mind enters tissue engagement and stimulates expansion. Expansion is the ultimate involuntary movement: it has no recovery phase, no active or passive phase, and no alternating contraction and relaxation.

Expansion is the involuntary response of the organism to overcoming gentle engagement through a continual dispersion of energy, a process appearing to have no end.

Expansion is prerespiratory. Although we might use the softening effect of the breath, its four mechanical phases can be distracting and disturb the flow of expansion. The deep

Chapter 5

expansion that wells up for an inhalation is phasic and differs in sensation and scope. Uninterrupted expansion is a continuous, nonrhythmic expression of energy, is beyond extension or elongation, and has an intimate relationship with consciousness. Unfettered consciousness is also expansive, and it has no acquired tension other than the tension of its existence. The material tension of tissue and the nonmaterial tension of consciousness interpenetrate through expansion.

Living tissue pulsates in a rhythmic combination of contraction and expansion. Antonio Damasio suggests that consciousness pulsates and moves in waves (Damasio 2000). It is said that the universe is expanding in order to overcome the wavelike pull of gravity. But aspects of practice demonstrate that expansion predominates as it overcomes physical engagement and mental condensation. Expansion is an expression of the entire organism reflected on its surface. Expansion is an ongoing, organic, emotional, and spiritual experience.

Expansion is a nonpulsatile, prolific, and pleasurable involuntary response to the tension of existence. Expansion radiates from a hub of engagement into the surrounding space, stimulating a parallel feeling of expanding consciousness and encompassing everything within its sphere of awareness.

The sleeve

On a microscopic level there are no fascial sleeves, but there are changes in the density of tissue. They appear and feel sleeve-like on a grosser level. The obvious sleeve, our essential guide and working tool, is skin and surface tissue. Skin has many

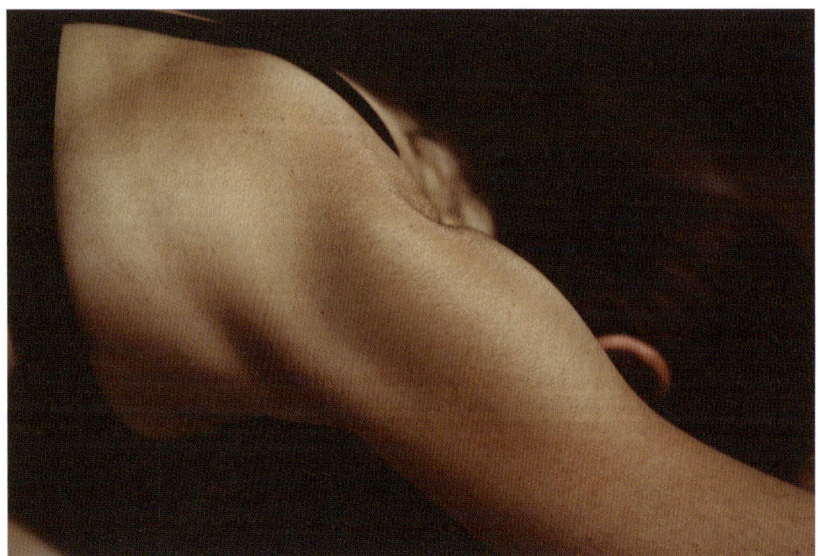

Expansion is an expression of totality reflected onto the surface of the body as an organic, emotional, and spiritual experience.

Sensing

more sensory nerve endings than muscle. We feel it move with the breath, and also when the breath is suspended. We can feel the surface move around and between the arms, pelvis, thighs, shoulders, and the circumference of the chest. We can feel skin move over the diaphragm, over the heart, and beyond. Permutations are endless as areas of skin relay movement in a myriad of configurations. The skin can also be felt as one continuous piece. Skin interfaces our inner and outer world, and is touched by the space that connects members of a practicing group. We are physically connected by the space touching our skin.

Neurophysiology divides the skin into areas called *dermatomes* that transmit information to and from specific areas of the spinal cord. Although this is useful clinically, every part of the cord knows what every other part is doing. Sensory conduction is also distributed through fascial networks, some of which may bypass the cord. However, in general terms one area of skin has access to the entire central nervous system. The skin is integrally woven into an outer layer of fascia which in turn is continuous with deeper structures. Moreover, the superficial fascia, lying just beneath and attached to the skin, is known to have a continuum of sensory distribution throughout its entirety.

The density of fibrillar tissue and the abundance or scarcity of sensory cells may be the factors giving us the feeling of layers within surface tissue. We are feeling changes in density. The terms epidermis, dermis, hypodermis, and superficial are terms of convenience related to function but they are basically one tissue. Movements of the epidermis, dermis, and hypodermis are continuous with one another.

The skin and superficial fascia resemble and can be *felt* as a body stocking facing outward and inward (its dark side). The surface is continuous with all deeper structures including the lining of the spinal canal, the spinal cord, and the periosteum surrounding bone and the internal structure of bone (Guimberteau & Armstrong 2015) and can be seen as an interconnecting skin investing and pervading all structures including the viscera. Our hearts and our skin are continuous. Surface changes and internal rhythms spread throughout the whole body as a consequence of tissue continuity.

The early embryonic unfolding of skin from a developing central nervous system establishes the skin's direct physical continuity with the brain. The outer layer of the brain, the cortex or rind, may be called the skin or sheath of the brain. The brain's encapsulating and divisionary membranes, the spinal cord, and radiating nerves are invested in skinlike sheaths that are continuous with the skin. All neurological and energetic functions resonate with the sensitivity and distribution of the skin. The body, brain, and skin are indivisible at the microscopic level. The three dermal areas – the epidermis, dermis, and hypodermis – and the superficial fascia are not only continuous over the body surface but also continuous with the deepest tissues. Therapies working with superficial tissue are effective on all levels due to the skin's deep connections. Nerve endings in the skin are highly sensitive to distortion and changes in tension, and particularly responsive to resistance and its release.

Chapter 5

> Lie on your back, with your legs over a bolster, and sense the finer aspects of your skin. Feel it move with the breath and between breaths. Follow skin sensation around the body from the chest and belly, down into your legs, up and around your shoulders, from one side of the body to the other and back again. Suspend your breath at the end of an exhalation, and sense the skin move with the fine involuntary pulsations of the deeper tissues. Take the group into this experience with you.

The skin is mapped on the brain and the brain provides the material base for the mind. Deane Juhan, author of *Job's Body*, describes skin as the outer surface of the brain and the brain as the deepest layer of skin. He writes:

The skin itself does not think, but its sensitivity is so great, combined with its ability to pick up and transmit so extraordinarily wide a variety of signals, and make so wide a range of responses, exceeding that of all other sense organs, that for versatility it must be ranked second only to the brain itself ... Nowhere along the line can I draw a sharp distinction between a periphery which purely responds as opposed to a central nervous system which purely thinks. (Juhan 1987)

His comments support the feeling that tissues have consciousness.

Nerves growing inward from the surface toward the spinal cord and brain have been instrumental in organizing the connections of the central nervous system. The organization of the brain is initiated at the surface of the body (Juhan 1987). This implies that a primitive mind, an ancient conscious awareness, began on the surface. The skin may unfold from central nervous tissue, but central tissue is in part stimulated and organized from the periphery. These discoveries explain the relationship between sensory suggestion and response. Sensory signaling, from surface to brain, has contributed to the evolution of consciousness. The skin has been instrumental in producing a mind.

The skin is no more separated from the brain than the surface of a lake is separate from its depths; the two are different locations in a continuous medium. (Juhan 1987)

A teacher can make suggestions based on involuntary activity. Involuntary tissue expansion and dynamic consciousness are not passive. As the mind empties, consciousness takes over, and tissue and consciousness expand together. Surface expansion also radiates inward. The action of the skin takes us deeply into the body–mind. Consciousness opens as skin opens, and skin opens as consciousness opens. Surface tissue is sensitive to our state of mind, dynamically responsive to our attention, and is the gateway to inner space and the realization that lies within.

Some areas expand readily, such as the fascial lining of the thoracic, abdominal, pelvic, and articular cavities. The surface is prolific. Centers of gentle engagement act as cores of

Sensing

expansion, and are particularly amenable to suggestion. The unbroken continuity of skin, its availability, and its inseparability weave into underlying fascia to make it the ideal organ of expansion.

It is relevant to understand that skin is the tissue of the ego. Alexander Lowen writes:

We thus have experimental confirmation of Freud's thesis that the ego in its perceptive function is primarily a phenomenon of the surface of the body. … One notes the absence of a muscular system … The ego is limited to the surface membrane. … At the same time it is the projection of the surface phenomenon [of the body] onto the appropriate area of the brain which makes perception as a conscious process possible. (Lowen 1958)

His observations, as with Juhan's, indicate the skin is the precursor to consciousness, perception, and awareness.

The skin is particularly responsive to touch, a primary factor in our evolutionary journey. The first contact of the infant's skin with his mother's skin gives an early sense of "I am." It is possible that "I am" may result from the earlier contact between the fetal skin and the *skin* lining the womb. Our skin gives us our sense of self. Further to this, Lowen writes:

On the psychic level, biological expansion is perceived as pleasure, contraction is unpleasure. … The movement of energy from the center of an organism to the periphery is identical functionally with biological expansion and with the perception of pleasure. (Lowen 1958)

As surface engagement opens pleasurably, its registration at the core relays back to the surface where it converts into further expansion. Expansion portrays the potential depth and scope of subjective experience. Expansion is equated with pleasure

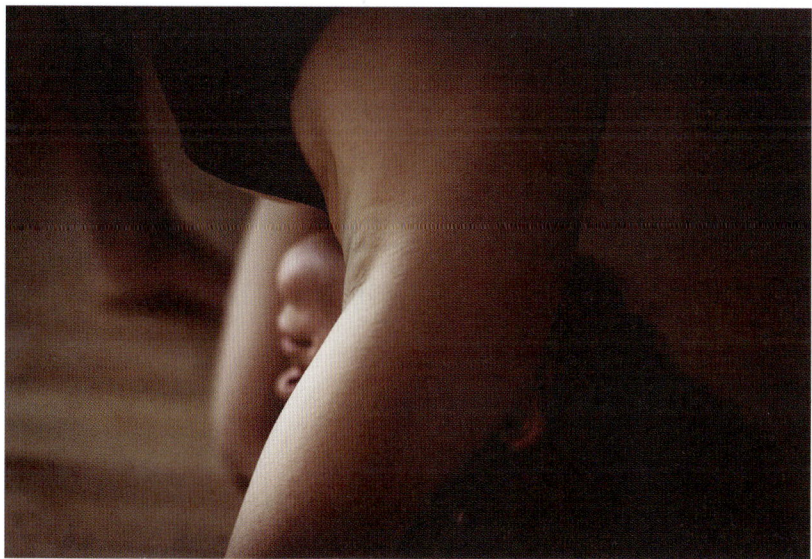

> Yoga begins when spatial consciousness places thought and sensation into perspective.

Chapter 5

and aligned with the expansive experience of spiritual bliss.

A continuum of space

Yoga begins when spatial consciousness places thought and sensation into perspective. Georg Feuerstein in his excellent book *The Deeper Dimension of Yoga* refers to King Bhoja, a tenth-century commentator on the Yoga Sutras, who observed that yoga is not so much "union" as "separation," and involves separating the self from nonself (Feuerstein 2003). In other words yoga puts space between the ego and something larger. Experiencing space in the body enhances mental space and the sensitivity needed to draw people out of their *selves*. Space frees the mind and reveals dynamic consciousness.

Spatial consciousness blends with the feeling of body space. Sensations of physical and mental space go beyond the sense of expansion and feed each other. According to Jean-Claude Guimberteau's research, based on microscopic observations of living human tissue, there is no empty space in the body. He observed

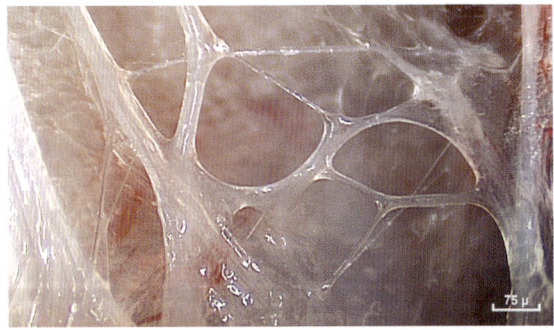

The fine texture of the fibrils that make up the microvacuole (Guimberteau & Armstrong 2015).

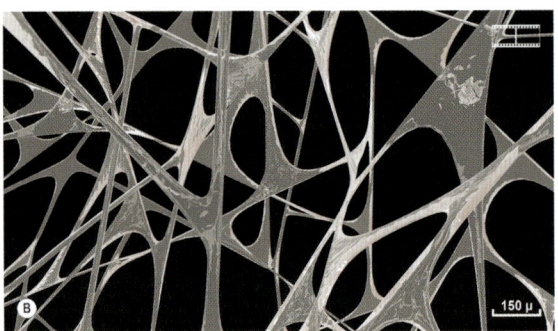

Hollow and cell-free spaces within fine connective tissue fibrillar structures (Guimberteau & Armstrong 2015).

numerous cell-free spaces but not empty spaces. The cell-free spaces are framed by intertwining fibrils and filled with substances essential to life. These cell-free spaces he calls *microvacuoles*, and they are revealed under traction and present a continuous web running throughout the body in all directions. His observations do, however, suggest that some fibrillar structures framing microvacuoles are hollow, and that microvacuoles generally lose their content under traction and only the fibrillar framework remains (Guimberteau & Armstrong 2015). Microvacuolar space is inhibited when traction exceeds acceptable limits.

The gentle traction of tissue engagement may contribute to our sense of space within the tissues. Fibrils also slide along each other in distinct separation zones. When the fibrillar framework moves, countless sensory nerves within tissue move with it, providing an uninterrupted supply of energy and information. This may give us our feeling of endless spread and expansion. At the microscopic level there *appears* to be no space between structures and no break in the continuity of connective tissue, but there are

SENSING

changes in densification. Spatial sensations may also arise from a dedensification. There may be greater sensory conduction where tissue has less density. Surface tissue has less density than the structures beneath it.

Guimberteau's compelling discoveries end where the atomic level of body space begins. The feeling of tissue disappearing may arise from an atomic or subatomic substrate. This may be where consciousness and sensation fuse to become a unified spatially dynamic *experience*. On an atomic and subatomic level, we are said to be 99 percent space, suggesting that basic units of matter comprising the human body contain empty space. This view is superseded by quantum physicists who suggest there are activities within the atom that suggest the presence of subatomic particles. There may be no such thing as completely empty space, just ever-decreasing densities without end.

The concept of space is relative to the density you compare it to. You can see why the yoga masters perceived consciousness as matter, as they endeavoured to dissolve their density. In this respect, consciousness and experience would have heaviness, hence the yogi's suggestion that ultimate bliss could only be found in the absence of experience.

There are a variety of spatial sensations that arise during practice:

- The feeling of actual space touching the skin externally. This sensation grows as the epidermis becomes more sensitive. External space is sensed by the tissue it touches.

- The feeling of space within the fabric of surface tissue during expansion, perceived as a separation of cells.

- We can feel surface tissue sliding around, which may be due to the sensory magnification of the sum total of countless microvacuolar fibrils stimulated by tissue engagement and expansion (involuntary traction). Tissues beneath the hypodermis (the superficial fascia) have a greater capacity for sliding. Their honeycomb arrangement is full of (relative) holes (Guimberteau & Armstrong 2015). Here again may lie our feeling of spread and space. Separation and sliding engages the entire surface, giving the feeling of interactive primary and secondary sensations.

- A feeling of space between the skin and superficial fascia and between the fascia and muscle. Changes in density may feel like relative space.

- A feeling of space between large segments of the body, between pelvis and thorax, thorax and cranium, due to their mechanical separation.

- A feeling of space within the pelvic and thoracic cavities which may be due to changes in texture and density and the proliferation or scarcity of sensory

Chapter 5

nerves as one tissue becomes another. The lining of the ribcage can be clearly felt, as opposed to its contents which need a stretch of sensory imagination. It does feel at times that we can feel the presence of our heart. Heart texture is responsive to attention.

- A sensation of space between the bones, within articulations, highlighting their shape and relationship.

- The spatial sensation of the dedensification of tissue coexists with the feeling of the decondensation of mental activity concerned with thought, giving space to the mind, consciousness, and experience (spatial consciousness).

- Space around and between group members.

- Vast inner space sensed as a gateway to the feeling of beyondness.

- Infinite space, sensed as a blending of an inner void with the space around us, as if we return to a time when only space existed. This experience touches on the research of quantum physics.

As far as we know, space has no awareness of itself and is free from conditioning. Space reflects the ultimate *isness*. An awareness of body space relies on the mental space needed for receiving the sensation. A soft inner margin can be sensed between the material self and an inner vastness free from conditioning and habit.

> Invite space between your sensations and thoughts. Put space around your total experience. Look at the possibility of tissue space merging with the space within and around you.

Space connects

King Bhoja must have known that the space separating small and larger selves also connected them. The space between elements of existence also unifies them. The space that pervades physical practice is interconnective. Space has structural, functional, and spiritual implications. Everything is connected by and through space. The feeling of solidity is illusory. The molecular structure of tissue and fluid is grounded in space. Space is the ultimate connective tissue connecting all things material and nonmaterial, cell to cell, tissue to tissue, density to density, body to mind, and thought to thought. Space connects us to the stars.

There are two tendencies in early embryonic development: a connecting tendency and a space-making tendency. ... In the first embryonic week, only the dimension of space is present. (van der Wal in Stirk 2015)

We can cultivate space between response and action. The space between us also connects us. In cultivating the separational aspect of space we connect more intelligently. Our physical, emotional, mental, and spiritual aspects thrive when given space. Space is free from personal history, beliefs, or ideas. Space does not interfere. Space provides the fertility for existence, it unifies, has no agenda, and is *the* spiritual

SENSING

common denominator. The space within and around us is continuous with infinite space.

Our natural state of being is relationship, a tango, a constant state of one influencing the other. Just as the subatomic particles that compose us cannot be separated from the space and particles surrounding them, so living beings cannot be isolated from each other … this tango extends to our thoughts as well as our bodily processes. (McTaggart 2003)

> As you open to expansion, invite a sense of space between and beneath the cells. Feel the continuity between the space above and beneath any given area. Local space is undifferentiated from the space beyond us. The effect on consciousness is revealing and extraordinary. Body consciousness and mind consciousness belong to limitless space.

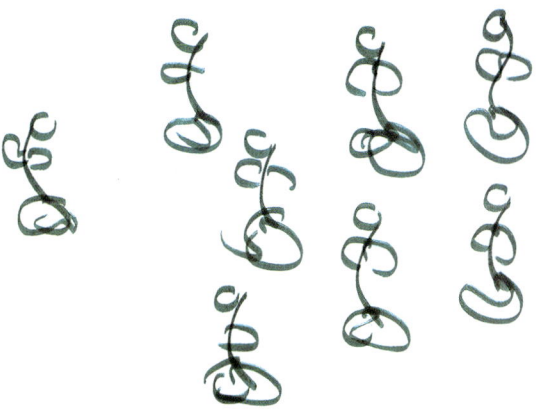

Space separates and connects all things material and nonmaterial. Space is the ultimate connective tissue.

Hovering

When we hover, we *hesitate before taking action and suspend our attention over or about a particular spot*. The art of sensing space begins by hovering over engaged areas and giving consciousness time to adjust to the sensation. The external space touching the skin is alive with energy, acting as a contact point from which to enter the tissue. The mind can then enter tissue space and move inward while maintaining a spatial relationship outside the body. We can sense outer and inner space as one coextensive space separated by a delicate membrane: the skin.

Iyengar made the following comments on space: "The final element that corresponds with the final sheath of bliss is called 'space' and allows mobility and freedom in all others. Space is the most subtle and pervasive element, and we must learn to tame it" (Iyengar 2005).

Here Iyengar refers to the emptiness of atoms, gleaned from the information available to him at the time, and based on his own experience:

Space … is taken in its old sense as being the space permeating the emptiness between particles of matter. The amount of matter inside an atom is equivalent to a tennis ball inside a Cathedral, so our atoms, and therefore we, are almost entirely space. The spaces above us, the sky, is … (cosmic intelligence in space) while the Self within is … (cosmic intelligence inside us). One is the external space, the other is the internal space, but to yogis the felt space of the Self is actually larger than that of the external space surrounding them. (Iyengar 2005)

Chapter 5

He continues:

Earlier I related air to touch and to intelligence. I said we both inhale and bathe in it. Space is even more intimate, more pervasive, since all of our atoms are mostly composed of space. Sound and vibration correspond to space and can travel through them. (Iyengar 2005)

Felt space

Spatial sensations are not imaginary (but can be imagined). When tension disperses, tissue awakens and sensory nerves pick up information usually beyond their scope. Feelings of space within tissue come from its response to the lightest engagement. As tissue decondenses, we can feel an increased density of external space. As superficial tissue yields, we pass through into an impression of deep endless space surrounded by an encapsulating sleeve. This transcendent feeling moves the mind beyond its habitual patterns and dynamizes consciousness. We encounter the Eastern experience through the unification of external space, internal space, and consciousness blending with a sense of infinity.

Space within cavities is at first distinctive from surface space. Visceral structures have little proprioceptive possibility, and the linings of the pelvic, abdominal, and thoracic cavities feel like they surround emptiness. Articular space enters awareness from fascial and membranous tissues. We can sense space between skin and superficial fascia and fascia and muscle. Feeling the space between muscle and bone may be due to the sensory nature of myofascial tissue and/or the periosteum investing the bones. We also become sensitive to changes in density between tissues, as sensation in some areas awakens more than adjacent areas. Guimberteau's findings suggest that the fibrils of vacuoles divide into smaller fibrils under traction so that their energy is spread more efficiently. This makes sense experientially, as the sensation of surface energy spreads out from engaged areas into the entire body.

> Spend time in a posture. Look at the relationship between mental activity and expansion. Notice how excessive tension stimulates ego contraction and inhibits expansion. Look more closely, slow down your mind even more. Engage with pleasurable sensation. A hub of delicate engagement expands throughout tissue, consciousness, and space. Observe how expansion spreads out into a continuous and endless spatial experience.

The idea of space is not the experience but leads into the experience. Directive imagery widens and elongates the body. The idea of space does not necessarily have a linear direction but it can do (the back of the knee opens vertically and laterally). Suggesting length or width based on what we feel is at first helpful. But the space within expansion is multidirectional and *radial*. Space within the expansion of the thigh, thorax, or back of the waist opens *radially*. We can sense the space, that opens within tissue from between cells, extend into the deep body and also outward beyond its surface.

We can introduce (more) space beyond the body, suggest space between the body and

SENSING

floor, between one another, and between ourselves and the walls and ceiling. We can refer to space beyond the room, building, street, or city into infinity, because it's there! Space brings lucidity and calmness and enhances presence, tempers emotion, dissolves thought, and gives time for students to feel. Space puts all activity into perspective, opens and activates deeper consciousness, silently connects us, and reflects a sense of *knowing*.

We could suggest a scale of densities. Beginning with the *con-density* of conditioned thought and tissue, through to the *de-con-density* of spatial and dynamic consciousness, all experiences could be graded by the extent to which the ego holds on to them or lets them go. It could apply to the ongoing fact of experience, regardless of content. I once shook hands with a Vedanta monk who meditated for four hours a day and had been doing so for 30 years. His hand felt like the lightest silk, full of vitality.

> Lightly place your tongue on the roof of your mouth and sense the space between them as they unify into an ever-dissolving sensation. Follow the feeling throughout your cranium. Feel your cranial space open and receive space from your pelvic and thoracic space and blend with the space around you.

Through the lens

The density of conditioning interlaces with phases of lucid spatial consciousness. As space replaces each level of conditioning, another waits to surface. The conditioned nature of thought invades spaciousness. An ever-present interference exists at all depths because *we are there*. We take our *selves* into the process. Acknowledging spatial experience is also an interference. Surrendering all activity reveals a dynamic intensification of consciousness that cuts through all boundaries. We are organized around and within space. It passes through us.

> Take your mind into inner space and the space around you. Notice how mental activity creates a density that occupies spatial consciousness. Pass through all mental activity. Notice that a part of you operates from the condensation required for guiding others, while another part of you is an aspect of continuous space.

Body space and spatial consciousness are a collective sensation. Space enters consciousness as a sensation. The sense of *knowing* arises from a sense of inner space and frees the mind from conditioned perception. Neurologist and psychiatrist Viktor Frankl put it well: "Between stimulus and response there is a space … In that space lies our growth and freedom" (Frankl 1946/1959). Space addresses complexity and identification, unites physical and spiritual experience, and facilitates the manifestation of insight and wisdom.

Teaching how to sense and feel is an art requiring sustained sensitivity. Sensitivity thrives on space around the teacher's experience, around the student's experience, and within the space between teacher and students. Words are objects within a

Chapter 5

shared spatial consciousness. Space magnifies words. The words expansion and soften have more impact when isolated from other mental activity, when they are given space. Change occurs within the fertility of space. We cannot do or make space, it arrives.

Getting out of our own way is the starting point. The art of sensing and feeling is in learning how to sense and feel. Sensitivity is magnified by mental space. The silence of space is the lens through which the laser of consciousness peers into itself and into the body.

> Engage with a local sensation. Find and enter its center. You will discover there is nothing there as it disperses into empty space. Quiet, penetrative attention passes through physical delicacy into infinity.

Seduction

Sensation is the initial attraction. When was your last memorable experience? How many students came up and said "that was amazing" or "I felt that for the first time"? Sensation is seductive, and it brings us back to the floor time and again. Sensations include: softening, fluidity, gathering, melting, lengthening, widening, gravitating, lightness, expansion, and space. Expansion is particularly enlightening. It occurs around deep emptiness and opens the soul. We let the light in and let it out.

> Focus on your skin over and around a center of radiation. Pass through the center. Be aware of a mental shift as consciousness and skin follow each other into the space within and surrounding you. Feel the radiation permeate the room. Convey the experience.

It is satisfying to perform a back bend or forward bend with ease, to feel the sacroiliac joints move spontaneously, sense the craniosacral rhythm, and the unsolicited adjustments of the diaphragm. But it is transformative and transcendent to follow the expansion of sensation and consciousness.

Creative engagement is comparable to the potter's clay, as we mold ourselves and those with us into an ever-subtler sense of self. Space is the ultimate freedom. Life has materialized from space. We return to our spatial origin.

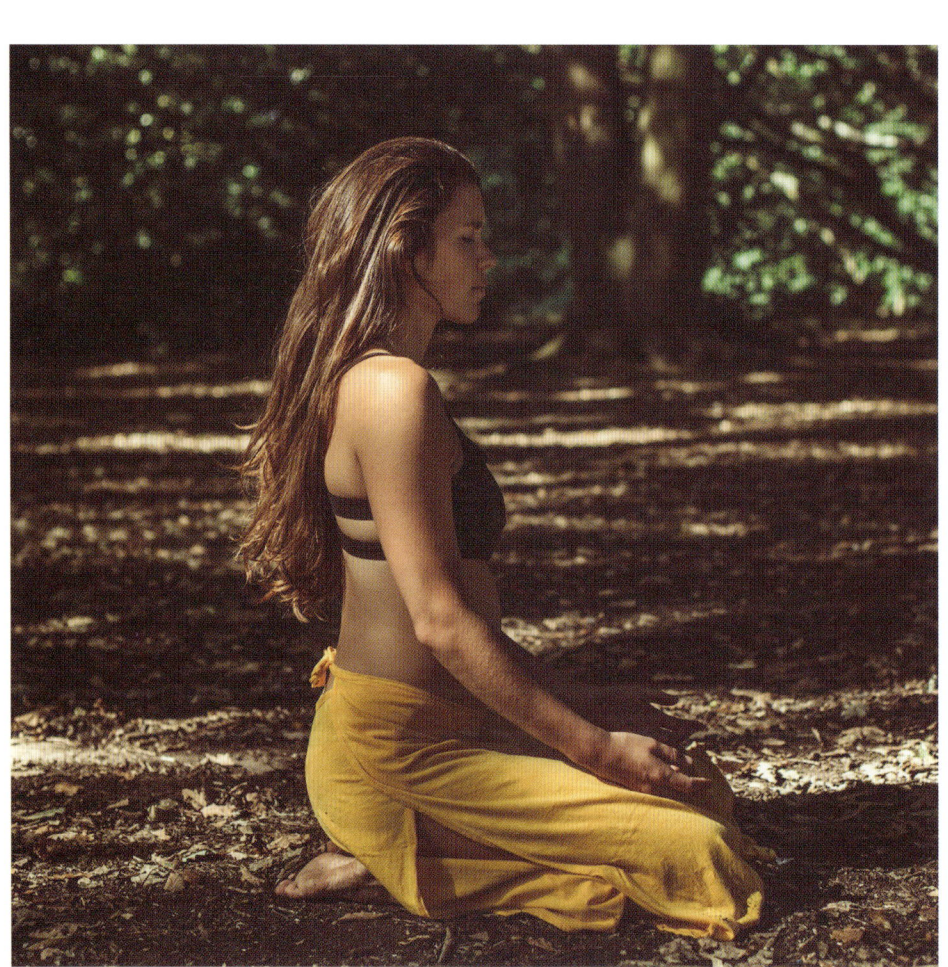

FIELDS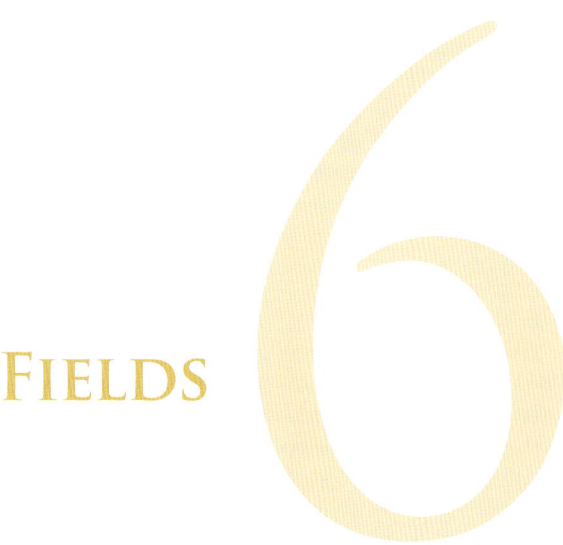

Something happens in groups, which has an intensity more profound than an "atmosphere." Are we tuning in to or producing a "field?" Experiences of this kind have resonated as a phenomenon of interest to physicists for a century or more and have provided practitioners through the ages with a basis for metaphysical philosophy and practice.

Fields of influence

The expression of living tissue and consciousness belongs to a universal field. *Fields* are defined as *nonmaterial regions of influence*. In physics, a *field* is defined as *the area or space under the influence of or within the range of some agent*. Taken literally, *influence* means *to flow in*. Fields are said to flow into, through and out of us. Transpersonal psychologist Arthur Mindell described a field as: "the atmosphere or climate of any community, including its physical environment and emotional surroundings. ... fields are natural phenomena that include everyone, are omnipresent, and exert forces upon things in their midst" (Mindell 1992).

Beyond William James's suggestion that the sublimity of individual consciousness accounts for the universal experience, the theories around fields are compelling: "Extra dimensions are no longer the preserve of esoteric speculations; they are mainstream, in modern physics" (Smolin in Sheldrake 2011). "But what do these extra dimensions do, and what difference do they make? Some physicists propose that they include 'information fields' that could help to explain the phenomena of life and mind" (Sheldrake 2011).

Field of fields

In her book *The Field* Lynne McTaggart writes: "Human beings and all living things are a coalescence of energy in a field of energy connected to every other living thing in the world. This pulsating energy field is the central engine of our being and our consciousness" (McTaggart 2003). She presents and examines research conducted by physicists who suggest a *quantum field theory (QFT)*. A *quantum field* is the primary field in nature.

The quantum field is said to overshadow the gravitational field which needs the

Chapter 6

density of matter to exert its pull. QFT proposes that space is packed with subatomic particles of energy containing information. Physical matter is also comprised of the condensation of field particles. According to Einstein: "Fields cannot be explained in terms of matter; rather, matter is explained in terms of energy within fields," which suggests that matter is energy (Sheldrake 2011). Pioneers of QFT proposed that space is brimming with activity, a vast primary field that contained and connected everything throughout the universe. They named it the zero-point field, suggesting it spreads out to connect all matter in the universe. McTaggart collates evidence of "an ocean of microscopic vibrations in the space between things." Fields are mediated by exchanges of energy. Field particles are knots of energy which emerge briefly and disappear back into the underlying field. Subatomic moving particles containing information spread out through space in a wavelike fashion. Space is an intelligence influencing our behavior.

Human beings and all living things are a coalescence of energy in a field of energy connected to every other thing in the world. This pulsating energy field is the central engine of our being and our consciousness, the alpha and the omega of our existence. (McTaggart 2003)

Based on her collated research McTaggart writes:

everything is a heaving sea of energy … living beings, including human beings, were packets of quantum energy constantly exchanging information with this inexhaustible energy sea. Living things emitted a weak radiation, and this was the most crucial aspect of biological processes. Information about all aspects of life … was relayed through an information exchange on a quantum level. Even our minds …

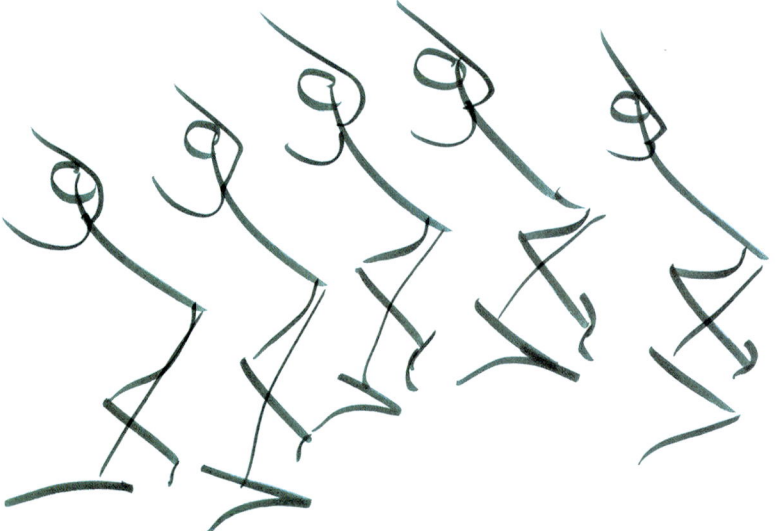

Space is an intelligence influencing our behavior.

FIELDS

operated according to quantum processes. Thinking, feeling—every higher cognitive function—had to do with quantum information pulsing simultaneously through our brains and body. Human perception occurred because of interactions between the subatomic particles of our brains and the quantum energy sea. We literally resonated with our world. (McTaggart 2003)

Quantum, meaning *amount*, describes, the lowest amount of physical energy that can be transmitted and exchanged. The *quantum field* involves the constant movement of energy. *Quantum physics* reduces all things material and nonmaterial to an indivisible connectivity and investigates the possibility of the absolute continuity of everything material and nonmaterial, a possibility suggesting that human consciousness has an extraordinary range. Antonio Damasio's theory that human consciousness arose from signals reaching the body from the external environment is overshadowed by the broader perspective of QFT. Whereas Damasio suggests that living consciousness needs an object from which to reflect itself (Damasio 2000), the quantum theory of consciousness resonates with Eastern metaphysics and attempts to verify an ancient belief that consciousness, not matter, is the ground of all being. Matter is secondary to consciousness. If everything is consciousness, we could be organic antennae, receiving and transmitting the energy of an infinite consciousness. Conditioning might represent waveband interference that disturbs reception. Penetrating the interference (the conditioning) tunes us to something infinitely greater than ourselves. Self, ego, and consciousness are made of invisible particles within an endless ocean of consciousness.

The idea of invisible unifying patterns inhabiting empty space supports a common group experience. Quantum theory resonates with the experience that consciousness is primary, and matter (the body) is secondary. Energy and consciousness spread out beyond the body filling the space around and between us. Eastern philosophy, and practice, has its scientific counterpart in QFT.

As each of us goes inward, intensifying our personal field, the resultant *coming outness* may contribute to the group field. Personal and group fields enhance each other. We may transmit sensation to others through a sensory field. A sea of energy may carry sensation and consciousness between us. In group work it feels as if the space between us is alive and connects us as a unified body. Together we *decondense,* a feeling of materiality melding with the nonmateriality. We touch on the unification of tissue sensation and infinite space.

Biological scientist Rupert Sheldrake in his book *The Presence of the Past* writes: "this way of thinking leads us back to the primal morphic field of the universe as the ultimate source and ground of all the fields within it. In the context of modern evolutionary cosmology, this is the original unified field from which all fields of nature were derived as the universe grew and developed" (Sheldrake 2011).

Seeing ourselves as condensations of energy with infinite connectivity resonates with our experience. It can *feel* as if our tissues are part of a grand unified consciousness and therefore *have* consciousness. We discover that an objective, ego-driven approach inhibits the fluidity needed for the "possibility" of informed energy to connect us, pass through us, and enhance a transcendental experience.

Chapter 6

The primary field is said to be infinite and unbounded. It provides the substrate for everything known and unknown, forms a basis for all possibilities, and pervades things material and nonmaterial, suggesting that materiality is in essence nonmaterial. The body is seen as the physical messenger, a condensed expression of infinite consciousness. Our palpable, seeable materiality is a representation of our nonmaterial nature, experienced as one energy at varying densities. We feel our tissue and selves as energy. This potential invites an emergent insight that *materializes* when thought is absent and tissue opens into surrounding space.

A theory

Theories suggest a ground substance of all existence, and its possibility for transmitting information across space and between organisms. Physicist David Bohm considered the organization of physical particles, living organisms, and minds in terms of a hierarchy in an undivided process of flux. This flux is made up of particles resonating with surrounding space and transforming into waves.

A teacher's sensation might be the vibration of particles travelling as waves: to become thought particles; to become waves that become spoken word particles; to become waves that become thought particles of group members; to become the waves producing the particles of their sensory experience.

If nonmateriality and materiality meet at a subatomic level, the following proposals are of interest:

- Matter and energy have wavelike and particle-like characteristics.

- Subatomic particles have a wavelike nature that spreads out through space.

- Fields are mediated by exchanges of energy.

- Particles are little knots of energy which emerge briefly and disappear again back into the underlying primary field.

- Every exchange of every particle radiates energy.

- Particles cannot be separated from the space that contains them.

- For matter to be stable it depends on a dynamic interchange of subatomic particles with the primary field.

Perhaps these theories shed light on the group experience of condensation and decondensation. We cannot feel the minutiae of the science at this level but can feel the spatial exchanges and energy within and beyond the body and between ourselves. We can share the possibility that the contents of space transmit information that connects us to each other and our environment. We can feel the *thickness* in the room.

The rigorous determinism of classical mechanistic theory softened into a science of probability. And spontaneity reemerged in everything. Even the vacuum ceased to be an empty void; it became a seething ocean of energy, producing countless vibrating particles all the time and taking them back again. A vacuum is not inert and featureless, but alive with throbbing energy and vitality. (Sheldrake 2011)

A field of consciousness

There is a limited understanding of what consciousness actually is or how it comes about. Rupert Sheldrake acknowledges science's lack of an explanation. He writes: "brain scanning and computer modelling have failed to explain the nature of minds, and in consciousness studies there is no agreed solution to the 'hard problem,' the very existence of consciousness itself" (Sheldrake 2011).

We can find inspiration in Krishnamurti's subjective experience: "When you become aware of your conditioning you will understand the whole of your consciousness. Consciousness is the total field in which thought functions and relationships exist" (Krishnamurti 1969). William James, over a century ago, recognized a "field of consciousness" as described by the psychologists of the day, who proposed that this field, seen as the entire contents of consciousness at any given time, had no clear outline. Its attraction is found in its unknown and potentially infinite range. James suggested fields within fields, fields overlying fields, and narrow and wide fields. The wider field implied an expansion of consciousness: "Usually when we have a wide field we rejoice, for we then see masses of truth together, and often get glimpses of relations which we divine rather than see, for they shoot beyond the field into still remoter regions of objectivity, regions which we seem rather to be about to perceive than to perceive actually" (James 1902/2018). James's observation resonates with the experience that "consciousness is a movement." Consciousness is marginless with an infinite range and in the absence of conditioned thought has immeasurable space.

Consciousness may elude scientific understanding, but all agree that consciousness is energy. If energy is a field then why not consciousness? Over the centuries yoga practitioners have understood consciousness subjectively, immersing themselves in its field and acknowledging its potential for radical transformation. Consciousness above all else is an experience. We can *feel its flow* within, around, and between us, as a profound and expansive sensation, moving out beyond the body, and coming from far away. Consciousness has a *texture* that can and should be cultivated. Pure unconditioned consciousness arises during focused attention on sensation and on consciousness itself. William James suggested that a field of consciousness "lies around us like a magnetic field, inside of which our centre of energy turns like a compass needle, as the present phase of consciousness alters into its successor" (James 1902/2018). Consciousness unfolds!

> At the height of group resonance explore the nature of consciousness. Refer to its texture, its permeating and connective nature. As tissue sense dissolves, highlight consciousness as the predominant element.

Consciousness may not be an exclusive property of brain neurocircuitry and

Chapter 6

biochemistry. The brain might be a generator and a condenser of consciousness fed by the environment. For the mind to exist it may depend upon a broader field of consciousness, with the brain as the organizer, as it tunes into the wavelength of a primal field. We might leach consciousness from all around us. The field theory attempts to provide the science behind the metaphysicality of Eastern beliefs. Prana and chi represent the grand fabric of a universal or global energy field that can be absorbed, experienced, and manipulated by living body–minds. We could be playing our part in an expansive and infinite consciousness. No one, as yet, has disproved theories proposing a *living* universal energy field from which consciousness can spread.

Einstein recognized that matter itself was "extremely intense," a disturbance in a sense of perfect randomness, and the only fundamental reality was the underlying entity – the field itself. The primary field is a repository for all fields and all the ground energy states and all virtual particles – a field of fields. Every exchange of every virtual particle radiates energy (McTaggart 2003).

Based on QFT the following may resonate with our experience:

- Mind and tissue belong to one field of consciousness.

- When you get down far enough into the quantum world there may be no distinction between the mental and the physical. There might not be two intangible worlds, only one – the field and the ability of matter to organize itself coherently (Jahn in McTaggart 2003).

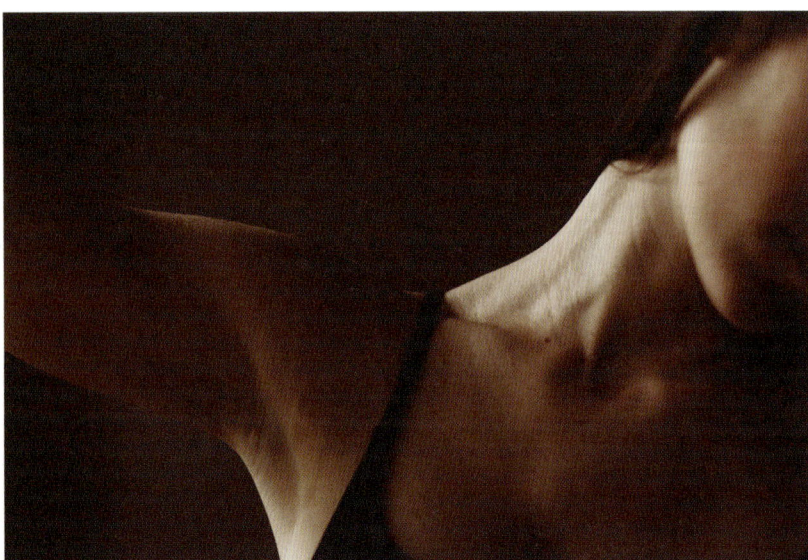

The brain might be a generator and condenser of consciousness, fed by the environment. For the mind to exist it may depend upon a broader field of consciousness, with the brain as the organizer, as it tunes into the wavelength of a primal field. We might leach consciousness from all around us.

- A field of consciousness is implicit in our energy field; it spreads out interweaving with everything around and beyond it.

- Personal consciousness and infinite consciousness differentiate out of each other.

- Consciousness is silent communication.

- The interconnectedness of everything softens our boundaries, drawing our individuality into a unified feeling.

A morphic field

Rupert Sheldrake introduces the concept of a "quantum body" communicating through a *morphic field*. Morphic fields are seen as fields of information by the quantum physicists. He writes: "In contemporary biology, one of the most promising ways of thinking about the development of living organisms is in terms of organizing fields, called morphogenetic fields. However, the nature of these fields has itself remained mysterious." He continues:

the nature of things depends on fields, called morphic fields. … Such fields shape all the different kinds of atoms, molecules, crystals, living organisms, societies, customs and habits of mind. … If we adopt an organismic rather than an atomistic perspective, there seems no good reason why organisms at all levels of complexity should not have characteristic fields. (Sheldrake 2011)

Sheldrake's proposition implies that individual traits and acquired or practiced ways of being can affect those within their field of influence. Group practice may draw on morphic fields. Sheldrake is unclear as to exactly what morphic fields are or how they work, although the concept is widely used in biology. He acknowledges that the physical reality of morphic fields is an assumption, but suggests that the body's tissues develop from a field that is as real as gravitational, electromagnetic, and quantum fields, and proposes the possibility of many more fields than those currently recognized by physics.

Fields suggested by morphic field theory might exist within the primary field of QFT. "The relationship of morphic fields to quantum matter fields is still obscure, but if they are similar in kind, not only would their interaction be easier to conceive, but a unified theory could ultimately embrace both" (Sheldrake 2011). Sheldrake suggests that for a unified theory of quantum and morphic fields to emerge, living organisms and conscious minds must be included. The morphic field would in all probability lie within the primary quantum field.

Spiritual teachers considering these theories might suggest that fields flourish in the absence of separative conditioning and propose that unconditional universal love is the consequence of a unified morphic or quantum field. As we feel into our experience, the idea of a quantum or morphic field may or may not cross our minds. I certainly refer to it in group work. More to the point, having accepted field transmission, what might the space between us be capable of transmitting, and to what extent does the quality of our presence as teachers influence transmission?

Chapter 6

Do we conduct sensory intelligence and an alternative consciousness? It feels as if we do!

Morphic fields may transmit biological information. "For example, an organ field organizes tissues, a tissue field organizes cells, a cell field organizes ... the nucleus and the cell membranes." Higher level fields may act on and modify lower level fields (Sheldrake 2011). Biological, mental, and emotional behavior are indivisible. If biological information can be transmitted then why not pleasure, dullness, confusion, excitement, knowing, awakening, and a consciousness free from content? An emotional field organizes emotions, a field of attention organizes attention, and a field of deep interest organizes deep interest.

The morphic fields of perception, behavior and mental function are rooted in brain activity, but they are far more extensive than brains. ... the fields of perception and behavior are intimately related to the activity of the brain, but they extend far beyond it, directed by attention and intention. (Sheldrake 2011)

The personal field

The morphic field is thought to shape our organism, but our development is also affected by genes and environmental influences. A field's quality is influenced by hereditary factors and conditioning. Each one of us has a field pattern that influences our behavior and way of being. It spreads out influencing surrounding fields. Research collated by Lynne McTaggart converges on a single point: "the self has a field of influence on the world and vice versa" (McTaggart 2003). Each of us has a two-way field that emits and receives from beyond our body. Each of us radiates a field with an intensity that changes from moment to moment depending on how we feel, the texture of our sensations, and the quality of our consciousness. Our boundaries move beyond the skin.

Energy scientist James Oschman writes: "the state of consciousness typical of those who practice meditation and yoga, is likely to entrain his brainwaves with the micropulsations of the earth's field" (Oschman 2000). A person is a total field made up of interwoven fields. Studies collated by James Oschman demonstrate various measurable fields emanating from the heart, organs, tissues, the brain, and consciousness. "It is a fact of physics that energy fields are unbounded. The bio-magnetic field of the heart extends indefinitely into space. While its strength diminishes with distance, there is no point at which we can say the field ends. ... it gets weaker and weaker until it becomes undetectable in the noise produced by other fields" (Oschman 2000).

Oschman demonstrates that the heart's radiation is greater than the brain's. Maybe this is because the heart does not think. Love is more potent than thought. Thought is a condensation of energy, while love is expansive (unless one has loving thoughts and even then the heart is in charge). As tissues expand, the ego boundary of the skin dissipates. Energy moves out from within, moving between and through us. James Oschman points out that any movement of any part of the body is "broadcast" into the space around the body as a signature of that movement.

Fields

Expansion is a large surface movement and we can feel its energy move out beyond the skin. The intensity of personal fields varies. Egos, selves, and minds behave differently within the field of consciousness. Excessive identification may inhibit radiation while relative emptiness enhances it. This is made obvious by the power of radiating consciousness emitted by some spiritual teachers.

The field of a teacher's presence acts upon the group, the group's field acts upon the teacher, and the field of each person in the group acts upon the others and on the group as a whole. One person's energy can affect the group, and there are differences in the fields of those who practice together regularly, compared to a group whose members are unfamiliar with one another.

The group field

A group with a unitive focus creates a local field of consciousness. Each word and its timing is inspired and evoked by group consciousness. People remark: "when you mentioned that, I was feeling (or thinking) it as you said it." Individuals, and often the group, can have an experience at the moment we experience and articulate it. Collective experience may be the sum total of personal fields. Personal sensation and consciousness create a mutual field. Larger groups with a heightened sensory awareness can have a deeper experience due to the strength of the field.

It might feel as if the group morphs into a cohesive unit manifesting as a singular organism, as if individuals replicate the cells of an organism. We feel, sense, *know*, and transcend together. Cohesion moves in

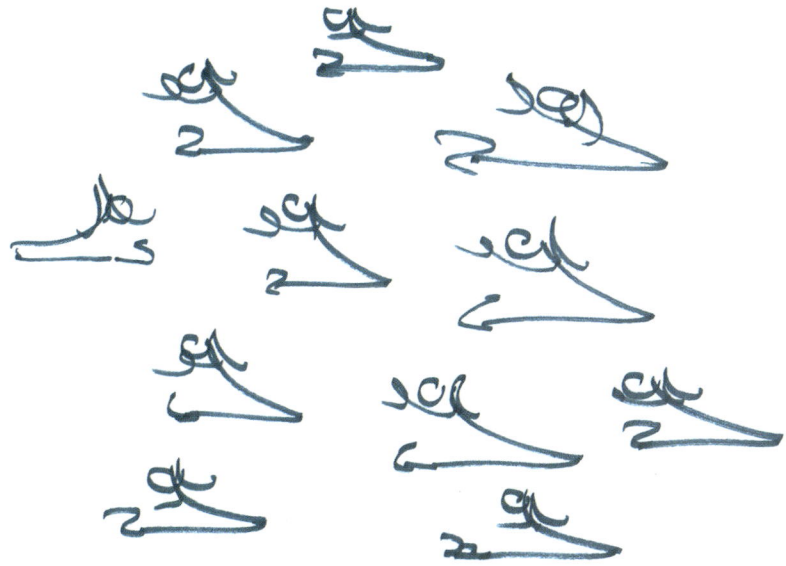

A group with a unitive focus creates a field of consciousness. A teacher's words, and their timing, are evoked and inspired by group consciousness.

Chapter 6

both directions, with each person radiating energy and absorbing it from the surrounding field. Individual minds contribute to a group mind and collective mentality. Freud suggested the collective mind was transmitted unconsciously. In our work, the intensification produces a conscious transmission because we directly address consciousness. Each person exploring a sensation, acknowledging spatial consciousness, and sharing the same silence binds the group into a field of purpose.

What these thoughts were leading up to was a model of consciousness that was not even limited by the body but was an ethereal presence that trespassed into other bodies and living things and affected them as if they were its own. (Braud in McTaggart 2003)

Researchers have designed machines that establish the presence of a field of consciousness during periods of peak group attention. "What appeared to be happening was that when attention focused the waves of individual minds on something similar, a type of group quantum 'super-radiance' occurred which had a physical effect" (McTaggart 2003). This happens in virtually every workshop I am involved in.

Research also shows that *need* enables greater access to the primary field. A group with the common purpose of feeling good, learning more, and going deeply is more open to the possibilities presented by field transmission. Although a field of consciousness provides a fertile space needed for the emergence of new experiences, these experiences may be subject to conditioning as they enter awareness. New experience may be filtered through a screen of previous experience. The strength of the group field acting upon each person softens and dissolves personal conditioning, and in turn reinforces group consciousness and cohesion.

The research presented by McTaggart, Sheldrake, and others provides a scientific theory supporting group experience. The transformation comes from direct experience! We can *experience* fields of consciousness and sensation. Expansion travels and fields connect us. Deeply focused attention to the body and to consciousness dissolve the barriers between individual condensation and the feeling of *something more*. Carl Jung was cautious of the collective power of groups. He felt the route to world change was based on individual self-reflection and the return of the individual to their own deepest being (Jung in McLynn 1996). Today group practice is more favored than

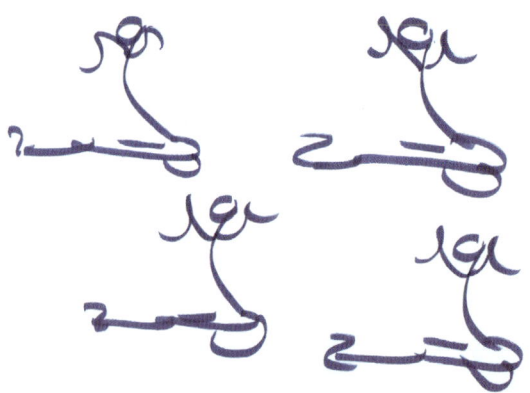

The strength of the group field acting on and with each person enables the dispersion of personal conditioning and in turn reinforces group consciousness and cohesion.

Fields

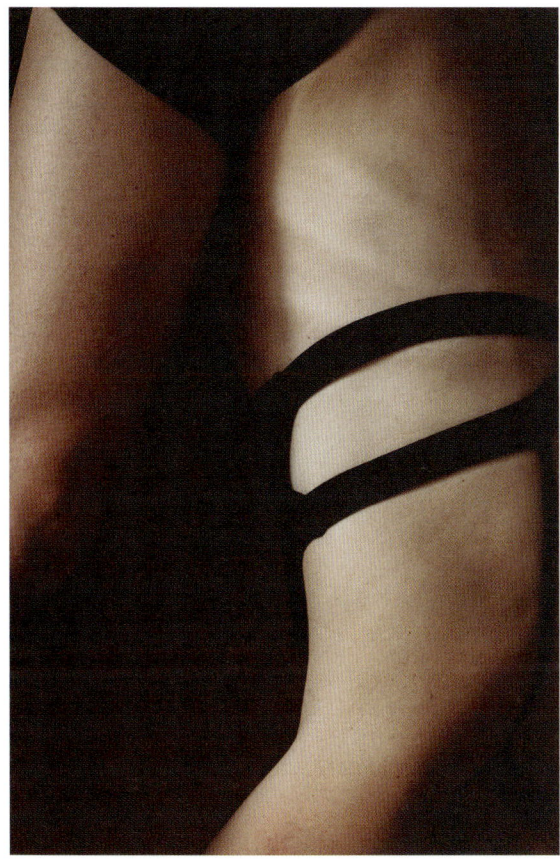

A teacher's field merges with the group field to dynamize the space and draw out collective consciousness. We hold and stimulate the group field by acknowledging the presence of the field itself.

ever. With respect to Jung's point, we can return to the core of our individual being *collectively*. Personal and group fields feed and deepen each other.

The teacher's field

The influence of a teacher's field involves various factors. Inspiration is essential and relies on our discoveries and current understanding. *We have to share it.* Just as important is our quality of presence, which is as relevant to the depth of a session as its content. *Presence* is defined as an *embodied self.* Presence is a sensation. Although we obviously "feel" present, the feeling is highly charged in a group and drawn out by the group field. A quiet, subtle tension, a fluid sense of understanding, radiates from teacher to group. Presence is also defined as the state or quality of having one's wits about one, calmness in exacting circumstances, and freedom from embarrassment, agitation, or panic. Depth of presence comes from an undisturbed inward and outward movement of awareness producing a generous and sensitive sense of self. The center of radiating presence is found where the inward movement (of oneself) unfolds into an outward movement (of oneself).

A teacher's field merges with the group field to dynamize the space and draw out a deeper collective consciousness. We hold and stimulate the group field by acknowledging the presence of the field itself.

Sense the surrounding field, draw the group's attention to it, bathe collectively in its density, and immerse yourself in the field experience.

Yoga as a culture has survived over centuries and is now in the ascendancy. Sheldrake suggests that cultural morphic fields might activate groups across space and time. As we

Chapter 6

touch the depth of our experience we can feel as though something comes through us from another time and place. This experience might indicate a connection with an ancient phase of ego development, or we may be channeling someone from the past! Have we been there before?

The intensification of a teacher's consciousness is transmitted to others. Research shows that people meditating together have highly synchronized brain patterns. Brains adopt the wavelengths of other brains. The person with the most coherent brain wave patterns supports and directs group energy and group consciousness. We can nurture a group before words are spoken, and during the space between the words.

Research (as well as our direct experience) shows we can influence the sensory possibility of others by our field. Some people are more receptive than others, and the nature of the work determines the outcome. Lynne McTaggart, during her research on the results of experiments on group consciousness, noted: "it was like a secret labyrinth that certain people could manoeuvre around more easily than others." McTaggart also refers to the research conducted by psychologist and behaviorist William Braud who discovered that it only seemed to work when he used gentle wishing rather than intense willing or striving. The relaxed passive receptive world of the field got results (McTaggart 2003). Braud's work led him to ask: if we can affect our own bodies through attention, can we create the same effect in others?

Spiritual guides consciously use their personal field to engage the energy of their audience: the stronger the presence, the deeper the effect. We can tune into presence before physical focus begins and invite everyone to join us by drawing attention to the *fact* of personal and group presence. We can start as we intend to finish, with an appreciation of consciousness and its field. Presence ignites the penetrative consciousness required to break through veils of conditioning. A teacher's presence stabilizes the group and reminds each person of their essential presence as they "take off."

> When your pelvic tissues are in expansion enter them with your entire field of awareness. Feel space within the tissues radiate out through the pelvis, giving it extraordinary lightness as if you have no pelvis, just space between the femurs and spine spreading up into your waist, chest, and neck, just the emptiness of space. Sense your personal field in relation to a vast interconnective field. We are an extension of universal space. It is an extension of us. A field of presence holds us in suspension.

A newfound sense of freedom requires a stable presence to support an excursion into what might be unfamiliar territory. The *presence* of presence is physically, emotionally, and spiritually grounding. We should be grounded in our own presence in order to remind others of theirs and support their experience.

The emotional field

We share a field of subtle and often palpable emotion. The emotional field should be acknowledged due to its power, range, and contagion. Emotion has a much older evolutionary vintage than conscious awareness. Endorphins, oxytocin, and adrenaline existed long before a sensory cortex could inform us of our emotional state. Emotions are body sensations. It is possible that, along with the broad range of sensations that contributed to an awakening consciousness, an emotional stimulus may have played its part. Perhaps all experience has an emotional charge, albeit at times an extremely subtle one. This may be why advanced practitioners thought it necessary to cultivate a nonattachment to all experience. Dispel thought, sensation, emotion, and experience and realize the ultimate freedom! A sense of complete freedom (from oneself) is impossible to sustain because it implies freedom from emotion, including the hazy elements of emotion highlighted by a deeper practice. We are attached (to one another) *by* emotion and therefore attached *to* emotion. The art would be in sustaining a sense of self, which is an experience, while enjoying a relative sense of freedom from oneself and one's emotions. The yogis attempted to sacrifice emotional attachment to others (the best kind) for the fluid emotion of altruistic love or even sustainable bliss. For us, life may have other ideas.

Emotion has great range but does not have the plasticity of ego–consciousness. It is more difficult to temper emotion than it is general behavior. The combination of emotion and conscious awareness has ensured human survival. The evolution of consciousness has enabled us to register and assess emotional activity passing back and forth on a more or less continual basis. Consciousness allows feelings to be known and thus promotes the impact of emotion internally. Consciousness allows emotion to permeate the thought process through the agency of feeling (Damasio 2000). We can be emotionally affected by the registration of an emotion, for example, fear of fear or joy at being joyful. Realization may be seen as an enlightened emotion, a flow of understanding.

We feel some but not all emotion. Aspects of emotion functioning beneath consciousness register in the deeper body–mind. Emotion is ever present because life expresses itself through feeling. Freud believed that the unconscious inner life was far more important than the inner life we are conscious of.

Basic emotions such as happiness, joy, fear, love, and anger are shadowed by a myriad of background activities containing an emotional charge. Background emotions are less well defined, but as awareness opens they are projected onto the screen of consciousness. Some are potentially obstructive and some constructive. They include pride, satisfaction, insecurity, impatience, expectation, disappointment, excitement, anticipation, pleasure, unpleasure, enthusiasm, calmness, or light heartedness. Anything that can be described as a feeling has an emotive substrate. Thoughts have an emotional content. A thought has a corresponding emotion and may be preceded by it. Distinctive thoughts may mask the emotions that precede them. All thoughts and emotions are responses or reactions *to something experienced*. This includes memory which recalls past experience.

Chapter 6

> During your own practice be attentive to all background activity as it passes through awareness. Notice the fine emotions that surface and accompany drifting thoughts and sensory acknowledgments.

Engaging surface tissue provokes thought and emotion and gives an opportunity to transcend both. Passing through thought brings background emotion to the foreground of awareness where it too can be transcended. "Some level of emoting is the obligate accompaniment of thinking about oneself or about one's surroundings" (Damasio 2000). A constant play of background emotion wells up from within, influencing personal and group field radiation. The body is an arena for emotions to play out their expression and serve their purpose. Damasio writes: "certain conditions of internal state engendered by ongoing physiological processes or by the organism's interactions with the environment or both cause responses which constitute background emotions … Background emotions … are richly expressed in musculoskeletal changes" (Damasio 2000).

We understand these changes through direct experience. Physical and emotional sensations change in concert with each other. Deeper practice invites a clear, unbiased look at background emotion. The emotive flux we see and feel in others is indicated by holding patterns, eye movements, facial expression, or a person's general timbre. Untoward effort or "not getting it," is tied to background emotion. We can address this by enhancing trust within a noncompetitive, level playing *field*. Emotional activity levels out when expansion is in ascendance.

Pleasant or unpleasant sensations are obviously emotionally charged. Pleasant sensations clearly promote positive emotions, address tissue texture, and pave the way for emergent insight. Pleasure is expansive, it gives access to all *fields* and enhances group communion. Unpleasant sensations have the reverse effect by creating anxiety, fear, or even panic which further exaggerates discomfort. Consciousness may penetrate mild discomfort but excessive discomfort is contractive, and causes a withdrawal from the surrounding field. One person "suffering with effort" transmits a ripple of disturbance throughout the group field. Emotional responses to deeper work are personal. Not everyone has the same emotion or intensity of emotion at the same time. We cast a broad net of awareness to acknowledge and support the variations in feeling. Each person in pleasurable expansion contributes to the harmonious emotional field in the room.

Tuning in to the emotional field requires presence and space. We hold the group in a way that enables emotion to process itself. The field of teacher and group provides a smooth transition through the unpredictability of emotion, thought, and sensation.

The unitive field

Consciously or unconsciously we are all comprised of the lowest common denominator – a condensation of connective field

Fields

energy. Energy is not conditioned but conditioning may either trap or leak energy. Consciousness and tissue arise from one energy. Physicist Renee Weber suggests that: "huge amounts of binding energy are needed to create and sustain the thinker and to maintain the illusion that he is a stable entity" (Weber in Wilber 1982).

Rupert Sheldrake identifies two versions of evolution. Evolution by natural selection and evolution by intelligent design fostered by an external intelligence. He quotes Henri Bergson: "the more we fix our attention on this continuity of life, the more we see that organic evolution resembles the evolution of a consciousness, in which the past presses against the present and causes the upspringing of a new form of consciousness, incommensurable with its antecedents" (Bergson in Sheldrake 2011).

Fields such as consciousness, attention, and sensation give and take from one another. At any moment sensation may become consciousness, attention may become pure consciousness, and so on. Any one field may occupy the foreground or background of awareness at any time, and any number of fields may be present at the same time. Each person in a group may tune into any one field, and all members may tune to one field simultaneously. At some point all fields may merge into one field of encompassing consciousness.

Consciousness holds us in a unitive field, consisting of the unconscious, the preconscious, basic consciousness, ego consciousness, group consciousness, collective consciousness, and whatever else may lie beyond. Fields of attention, awareness, interest, sensation, emotion, silence, knowing, and presence are enfolded within a unitive field of consciousness. Rupert Sheldrake writes: "there is nothing unscientific or dualistic about extended fields of influence pervading material bodies and reaching out beyond their surfaces. I suggest that minds likewise extend beyond brains through fields. Perceptual fields are morphic fields" (Sheldrake 2011).

If modern physicists in agreement with ancient practitioners are correct, and one field applies to the space and energy within and between all organic matter, our bodies and our consciousness can be seen as fields within fields. We and our tissues are connected by energy-rich space. We are inseparable from our environment. Rupert Sheldrake refers to experiments suggesting our self–body image resides outside the body. Are we downloading ourselves from the environment? Lynne McTaggart notes: "Each individual consciousness had its own 'particulate' separateness, but is also capable of 'wave-like' behavior, in which it could flow through any barriers or distance to exchange information and interact with the physical world" (McTaggart 2003). This can be experienced to a point during moments of deep, lucid awakening following the dispersal of all conditioned activity, as we (the group) appear to blend as one consciousness. Field transmission demonstrates a shared awakening.

Cores

Centers of sensation represent cores of energy radiating into the surrounding space and field. We may be conduits for a dynamic

Chapter 6

wavelength of living consciousness. We feel it in our bodies, in our minds, all around us, and in one another. Tuning into the wider field frees the energy of ego control and sows the seeds for creative insight.

Fields generally emanate from a core. The principle of *emanationism* refers to the theory that the universe emerged out of singularity, suggesting that all things are connected by a core of origin. We could see ourselves as a singularity in the process of decondensing. We emanate into the space around us. There may be as many cores as there are fields. Creative engagement is a radiating core merging with broader fields. Personal fields are cores blending with morphic and quantum fields. A teacher's presence acts as a radiating core, influencing the group.

The broadly accepted understanding is that consciousness arises from material brains. But if consciousness also has an external foundation, we may be its material conductor. Either way, our relationship to consciousness is accessible from either direction or both. The ultimate flow is captured in the following statement. "Even real particles are nothing more than a little knot of energy which briefly emerges and disappears back into the underlying field" (McTaggart 2003). Knots of energy are transient cores underlying conscious experience. According to quantum field theory, the individual entity is transient and insubstantial. In other words, particles (infinitely minute cores) cannot be separated from the space around them. It is OK to feel that consciousness is the consequence of spatial energy, although it may not be entirely proven.

Any *thing* can be a core. At one end of the scale the earth's mass represents the core of its gravitational field, and at the other end of the scale a living cell, or an atom, is a core of radiant energy. The core of a breath is found within the deep pause at the end of an exhalation. The spine is a mechanical core for the body, the brain the material core of mental life, and an idea is the core of an ideology. A method is the core of a practical approach.

We are defined by material density and nonmaterial behavior. The third lumbar vertebra represents a core of radiating gravitational energy throughout the body. Each spinal segment and each weight-bearing articulation is a localized gravitational core. Invisible gravitational lines identified by biomechanical principles are nonmaterial linear cores representing gravitational forces. The brain has a cerebrospinal fluid core within its cavities. The central nervous system represents a neurological core. The heart is the body's soft and expansive core. The density of every organ and tissue represents a material core of nonmaterial functional radiance. Organic substance radiates nonmaterial fields. Body cavities are functional organs expressing energy. Deep *felt* space within the thoracic abdominal and pelvic cavities radiates into surrounding tissue. A muscle belly is the core of the tissue surrounding it. Surface tissue is an expansive core, transmitting fields of energy between the deep body and surrounding space. Nonmaterial condensations of energy (chakras) are cores that are materially synonymous with corresponding neural centers. We consist of a myriad of interconnecting cores energetically resonant with one another and with the bigger picture. Personal consciousness is a radiant core connecting to a wider field.

FIELDS

> Look for a quiet and soft creative core of engagement spreading throughout the body into surrounding space, informing your behavior, mood, and realization. Your presence, feelings, thoughts, and suggestions are cores that produce fields of influence. Each person represents a contributing core. A focused group produces a core with a radiant field extending beyond its location.

As thoughts and sensations dissolve, the texture of consciousness and tissue changes with profound effect. Sensory experience normally perceives a distinct difference between substance and nonsubstance. Field theory suggests that every *thing* in existence has a physicality, including the space around us. Quantum physics and Eastern metaphysics highlight a confluence between materiality and nonmateriality. As sensation and sensitivity heighten, the delineation between material and nonmaterial substance softens and blurs. Nonmaterial aspects gain substance and bodies realize their spatial nature – *the lumbar spine blends with the space within and beyond itself.*

Traditional practitioners sought to transcend experience by passing through it. Experiences were seen as condensations (cores) of energy inhibiting the flow of pure consciousness. As they passed through each experience a subsequent finer experience manifested, and they passed through that. Sensation is a local experience acting as a core for a more expansive experience to be passed through again and again. The ever-enlightening core disperses the heaviness of experience to the point where we are *only just there*. We remain present but with a completely different texture. All experience is local because it belongs to the locality of

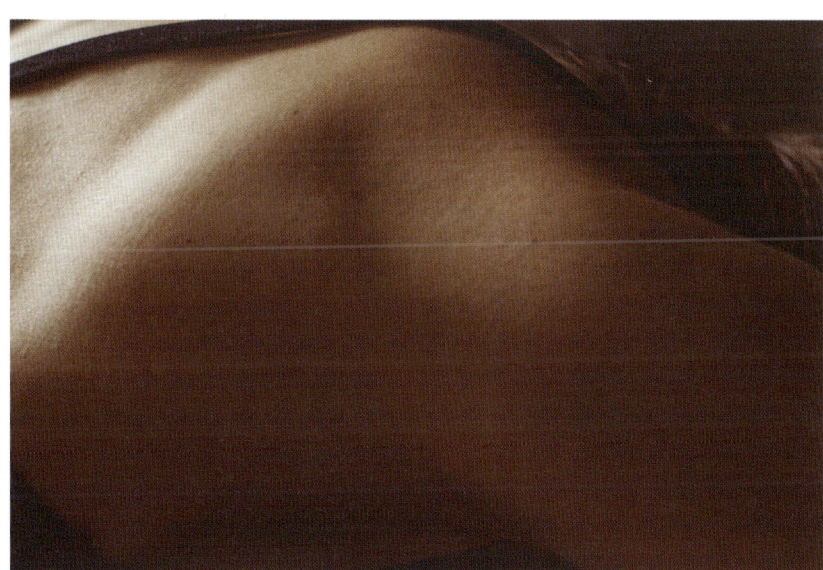

> We consist of a myriad of interconnecting cores energetically resonant with one another and with the bigger picture. Personal consciousness is a radiant core connecting to a wider field.

Chapter 6

the experiencer, but he feels he is somewhere else at the same time. We cannot get away from our experience entirely unless we are in a trance.

Constructive and obstructive cores

The consciousness of a teacher is a radiant core transmitting attention, awareness, sensation, *knowing,* and a sense of space. Experience has density, and all mental activity has substance. As we progress, we begin to feel the substance of nonmaterial experience.

Thought can be intrusive, heavy, and obstructive. Even the *recognition* of mental fluidity and spatial consciousness is a condensation. Transmission can be disturbed by an inappropriate remark, the sound of the breath, *doing* something in a particular way, or anything arising from a recondensation of the separative ego. If introduced at a sensitive moment, an obstructive core may be an idea on where a limb should be, a biomechanical principle, or an inauthentic spiritual soundbite. Obstructive cores have limited radiation. They are contractive, unyielding, and con*solidate* experiences.

Cores may be potentially obstructive to begin with but, once realized, can be lightened and dispersed by penetrative consciousness. A teacher may act as a constructive or an obstructive core. Good intentions can be either. Constructive cores are light, unheld, and dispersant. Light cores radiate with ease. Observations and suggestions are immersed in calmness and lightness and accompanied by gentle reminders that "this is just an observation."

Becoming the word

A thought or feeling may become a word. Students often have an experience as or even before our words conveying the experience are spoken. A field is at work. The tone and texture of our voice, choice of words, quality of presence before, during, and between words creates a field. On delivery, a word's meaning floats within space holding the group. Space, lightness, and consciousness are in the air. As our own experience manifests, we project condensations of mental energy with meaning (words) into the group experience. Words are projectiles to those in a state of sensitive transcendent awareness, hence the need to tread lightly and act slowly. For maximum effect, a word should permeate group experience, but it can disturb field interaction if its meaning cannot be experienced and released back into the field.

Physicist Renee Weber, in conversation with theoretical physicist David Bohm, noted that Bohm's contact with Krishnamurti had convinced him that familiar consciousness corrupts and therefore cannot reveal reality. She observed: "Thought is reactive and not an active ability, attuning man only partially to nature and distorting most of it. Thought is a fossilized kind of consciousness operating within 'the known' and thus by definition is uncreative" (Weber in Wilber 1982).

Weber's point invites a creative language that can address conditioned perceptions and point the way to the *unknown* of new experiences. If Krishnamurti and David Bohm had not shared their thoughts, we may have been unlikely to have received their insight. We seek the words that convey the message

FIELDS

even if the message may be partially lost by the use of the words. We can find appropriate language for sharing insightful thoughts.

The essential core

We are programmed for experiencing. Evolution is the consequence of experience upon experience, some beneath and some within awareness. Existence thrives on a core of experience. An *experience* is defined as *an occurrence which leaves an impression, something we undergo or have contact with,* or *a thought, fact, emotion or object*. We can *be* experienced *at* something or *have* experience. *Experiencing* is the subjective conscious awareness of our experience. We are continually subjectively experiencing and we fill our subjectivity with experiences. We are subject to and at the mercy of the ever-changing nature of our experiences. Experience per se is the essential core of conscious existence. The mystics understood that the quality of our experience is the key to an alternative consciousness.

The quality of our experiential nature is determined by the space afforded our experiences. It is found in the fertility of spatial consciousness.

Where does it go?

Where does the energy of an experience go to when the experience dissolves? Perhaps it returns to spatial experience before dispersing into the ether of no experience. An experience might be seen as a highly magnified representation of a quantum particle that disperses into a wave to condense again as the next experience and so on. An experience settles, informs, and disperses. Its dispersion determines the quality of spatial and dynamic consciousness. An insight might be an enlightened condensation of experiencing.

Yoga and metaphysics suggest a spatial core, central to all existence and personalized by an inner void of *infinite emptiness,* a nothingness that spawns realization. *Cores* in the form of physiological and philosophical concepts act as points of entry for opening spatial consciousness. *Information* can be absorbed, dynamized, and dissolved into space. If energy within space can transmit information, it follows that the less material the space, the more fluid the information flowing through it. Personal consciousness is a core of radiation within a broader spectrum of radiation. As soon as the *idea* of a broader spectrum takes hold, it becomes another core to be transcended. Experience is our essential core.

Closer to home

The impact of group work can also be explained by Freud's interest in group psychology. Freud did not refer to fields as such, but while recognizing that the herd instinct underpins group resonance, he pointed to the narrower circle of the family that sowed the seed for the group mind. The origins of group oneness may be closer to home. Individuals practicing together regularly can feel like a family.

Freud pondered that if groups have a unitive experience, there must be something

Chapter 6

to unite them, and there must be a group depth psychology. He wrote:

It is easy to prove how much the individual forming part of the group differs from the isolated individual, but it is less easy to discover the causes of this difference.

He noted:

… the lowering in intellectual ability which an individual experiences when he becomes merged in a group. … the notion of impossibility disappears for the individual in a group. (Freud 1921/1959)

Freud's observations show that the field of personal thought is weakened by group energy, making space for broader possibilities.

Freud frequently cites Charles-Marie Gustave Le Bon, best known for his work *The Crowd: A Study of the Popular Mind*, and McDougall, author of *The Group Mind*. Freud draws the following from their theories, comparing them to the depth psychology of psychoanalysis (Freud 1921/1959):

- "The feelings of a group are always very simple and very exaggerated. So that a group knows neither doubt nor uncertainty."

- "Anyone who wishes to produce an effect upon the group must exaggerate and must repeat the same thing again and again." This may also have a negative effect. A group leader may hold a group in sway, but if low on integrity or experience may impede the group's discoveries. This can happen without a teacher being aware of it and gives another reason for being in the experience with the group. A teacher's ego and group ego soften and dissolve together.

- "Under the influence of [positive] suggestion groups are capable of high achievements in the shape of abnegation, unselfishness, and devotion to an ideal. … It is possible to speak of an individual having his moral standards raised by a group."

- "A group … is subject to the truly magical power of words … 'as soon as they have been pronounced an expression of respect is visible on every countenance … By many they are considered as natural forces, as supernatural powers' … It is only necessary to remember the magical powers which they ascribe to names and words."

- "Momentous discoveries … are only possible to an individual working in solitude. But even the group mind is capable of creative genius in the field of intelligence, as is shown above all by language itself as well as by folk-song, folklore and the like. It remains an open question, moreover, how much the individual thinker or writer owes to the stimulation of the group … and whether he does more than perfect a mental work in which the others have had a simultaneous share."

- "The higher the degree of mental homogeneity, the more striking are the manifestations of a group mind."

- It is a pleasurable experience to surrender and become submerged in the group and lose the sense of the limits of

Fields

individuality. McDougall calls this: *"the principle of direct induction of emotion by way of the primitive sympathetic response"* – an emotional contagion (McDougall in Freud 1921/1959).

- *"There is no doubt that something exists in us which, when we become aware of signs of an emotion in someone else, tends to make us fall into the same emotion."* Insight and wisdom can be seen as emotions!

- *"Emotional ties constitute the essence of the group mind."*

- The greater the number of people, the stronger the overall effect. *"Something is unmistakably at work … to remain in harmony with the many. The cruder and simpler emotional impulses are the more apt to spread through a group in this way."* Emoting insight, wisdom, and amazement are good examples.

- *"The tendency towards the formation of groups is biologically a continuation of the multicellular character of all the higher organisms."*

- *"Groups are distinguished by their special suggestibility."*

- *"A group is clearly held together by a power of some kind: and to what power could this feat be better ascribed than to Eros, which holds together everything in this world?"* (Freud 1921/1959). This was Freud's personal acknowledgment of the power of love.

In Freud's terms a group practicing together has put the substance of the work and the person teaching it in the place of their separative ego. They have identified themselves with one another through the teacher. He points out: "We must conclude that the psychology of groups is the oldest human psychology. … Individual psychology must, on the contrary, be just as old as group psychology, for from the first there were two kinds of psychologies, that of the individual members of the group and that of the father, chief, or leader" (Freud 1921/1959).

Guiding groups into and through their individual experience enhances the group field as we tap into an ancient phenomenon echoing Jean Gebser's archaic and magical consciousness. Groups are suggestible and open to change, and depending on the approach the effects can be transformative.

The altruistic nature of our work and its potential for awakening consciousness cannot be overemphasized. We immerse ourselves and those with us into a field of possibility. Beyond the group each individual has the potential for processing their discoveries in their own way and time.

Other fields

If, as physicists propose, there are fields within fields, anything with a radiant energy (a single cell or a mood) has a field. There are many possible fields within group work that we can acknowledge as relevant, and there might be many more.

Chapter 6

The field of the ego. This is the starting point – personal egos contribute to the group ego. The field of the personal ego is separative until absorbed into the group ego by the nature of the work, the presence of the teacher, and their intention.

A behavioral field. Members of a group engaging in the same behavior create a field reflecting that behavior. As we blend into the depth and space of personal and group consciousness, internal behavior is softened, calmed, energized, and transformed.

A field of the voice. The tone, softness, depth, lightness, and intention of a teacher's voice creates a field within which others can access new discoveries. The voice can enhance or inhibit the presence of other fields.

A field of knowing. A group in tune with lucid consciousness at its most profound realizes an expansive sense of "knowing."

A field of love. As conditioning lifts, love arises spontaneously. Pleasurable sensations produce the intimacy of unsentimental group love.

A field of space. We feel as if we expand into space. An awareness of space predominates with the feeling that space has awareness. Everyone's inner space blends and unites within the space around us, as bodies decondense and the space around us condenses.

A field of silence. Silence is an intense form of communication. The stillness of silence inspires measured and considered speech. Silence between words places emphasis on what has been said and enhances mental focus. A carefully chosen word emanates from and is surrounded by silence. Silence is undisturbed by the appropriate choice and timing of words. Insight stems from a culture of silence. Authenticity is engendered by silence. The expansion of tissue and consciousness is the result and cause of silence. All activity is absorbed by silence.

A field of communion. We find ourselves in communion – a group spiritual experience without reference to spirituality. A spiritual field presides as consciousness opens. The feeling of "communing" is transformative.

The transcendent field. We pass through all activity into spatial and dynamic consciousness. We might be accepting the primary field of nature with a morphic field as the messenger. Dynamic consciousness disperses the group ego into a primary field.

The cosmic field. Cosmic intelligence has engaged the spiritual imagination for many centuries. "Cosmic intelligence is the organizing system of the Universe" (Iyengar 2005). The intensification created by the group field draws personal expansion into the bigger picture!

The remote field

The term *remote* may not be the most suitable term to describe the online trend. As well as *distant* the standard definitions of *remote* suggest: *obscure, having little connection to, detached* and *unrelated to*. But these definitions give little credit to the online experience.

The more appropriate definition of *remote* is *secluded*. Traditional practitioners would seek seclusion to minimize life's distractions. From the seclusion of their own homes each group member can use their attention as antennae connecting them to the teacher and to the group.

All fields are by definition remote in that they spread out. *Remote control* is transmitted through a man-made energy field. *Remote sensing* is a term used by science to describe the ability of technology to gather information about something.

Online work uses computer technology to *transmit* an experience. We transmit an organic experience that is picked up by students via their computers. A local organic expression is accepted organically "from a distance." Organic connections form the very beginning and the very end of the transmission. The technology *falls between* the teacher's and the students' experience.

There are two underlying spatial aspects to distance sessions. Firstly, the space that unites and pervades all things and secondly the cyberspace that passes through or surfs it. We connect through both. Cyberspace is supported by space as we know and experience it. Cyberspace is the computer mediated virtual world into which we plug our thinking and sensory minds.

The unifying factors that apply on-site also apply online. The group shares sensation, an alternative experience, and a potential shift in consciousness. Because of their "aloneness" each student feels that we talk directly to them, an on-site experience that is heightened online.

The absence of a live group gives an opportunity for refining our approach and developing our yoga voice. Online work lends itself to the quality and impact of speech. Beyond a point there is no need to *show* people what to do. You cannot *see* consciousness and sensation but acknowledging their combination cultivates an innovative way of working. We can creatively and productively enter and enhance the experience of others from a distance.

The online voice is essential and therefore more powerful. Its tone, rhythm, and meaning are amplified as we deliberately project and give voice to our own experience, repeatedly referring to sensation and consciousness in order for "yoga" to manifest.

Each word is not only a concept but also an image and an introduction to, or reminder of, a sensation and a way of being. *Sensation*, *consciousness*, and *field* are prime words implying a primal experience.

Sound is founded on a backdrop of silence. The sound of silence or the silent space between and beneath words is as fundamental to their meaning as the voice itself. The space of silence is cohesive, particularly if our imagination subscribes to the all-connective theories as put forward by quantum physics, field theory, and morphic resonance. Intervening silences give time for our words to "sink in," and become a shared experience.

The field of the voice and the field of silence coalesce to draw everyone into an ever-deepening alternative way of being. Some might say we are unconsciously

Chapter 6

(or consciously) reminded of the silence and seclusion of the womb, or the in-utero resonance of our mother's voice.

Basic elements unify teacher and group and deepen experience, for example:

- Common purpose and intention.

- The teacher's voice and presence providing the core of radiation.

- The teacher's feeling of "channeling" from another place and time is enhanced by the additional dependence on and embracing of the fields at large. This deepens and broadens group perspective.

- The profundity of intervening silences drops the group into their depth.

- A "remote field" unifies the group and sustains attention.

- Drawing the group's attention to the field presence.

- Inner spatial experience facilitates an acknowledgment of the geographical space between us.

- Remote participation adds to the sense of "an unknown element," upon which the entire yoga experience is founded.

- The teacher in turn is inspired by the presence and quality of the group's attention. Our field is strengthened. We know that they are *there* regardless of how we organize the screen.

If, as suggested by yoga masters, mystics, and physicists, we have descended from energy in space, and if we are organic condensations of our spatial environment, our deeper organic nature should be comfortable with returning to and transcending the space between us.

Remote teaching works and the response can be extraordinary. Emma had the following experience in the seclusion of her home 200 miles away.

A remote experience

"In last week's evening workshop I experienced something that has, as they say, both changed everything and changed nothing, but which I will hold and know for the rest of my life, a moment of pure acceptance and holy presence. It may have lasted seconds or minutes, I can't say because it was timeless. It was a moment of being utterly and distractedly alive (it was something holy – but liminal, sacred.) Other words will do. It was a religious experience, about the very essence of life and death and completely outside time. It was a moment of peace, of both such intensity and such emptiness. I feel I can never forget it, but never describe it."

On-site or online, the fertile combination of personal space, group space, and spatial and dynamic consciousness provides an opportunity for the materialization of deep insight and realization. The local and distal fields that we are a part of and create can be the source of enlightening and transformative experiences.

We are connected through and by space, the ultimate connective tissue, drawing all material and nonmaterial aspects of existence into a unified whole. We can indulge our penchant for "a universal experience" by entering into remote participation, each person acting as a satellite and forming a group field with the teacher at its center.

Resonant communication

What is the feeling as we sit quietly facing a group, seen or unseen? We feel the group and the group feels us. We sense into others while others sense us – the ultimate resonant communication devoid of voice, instructions, or suggestions. We sense others arriving into our body–minds as we enter theirs. Fields suit our purpose as we share dynamic space. Heightening a group's sensitivity and giving them the opportunity to transcend themselves from a distance is another kind of transcendence. It is a skill that is found deeply within our innate capacity for communication. A little love goes a long way!

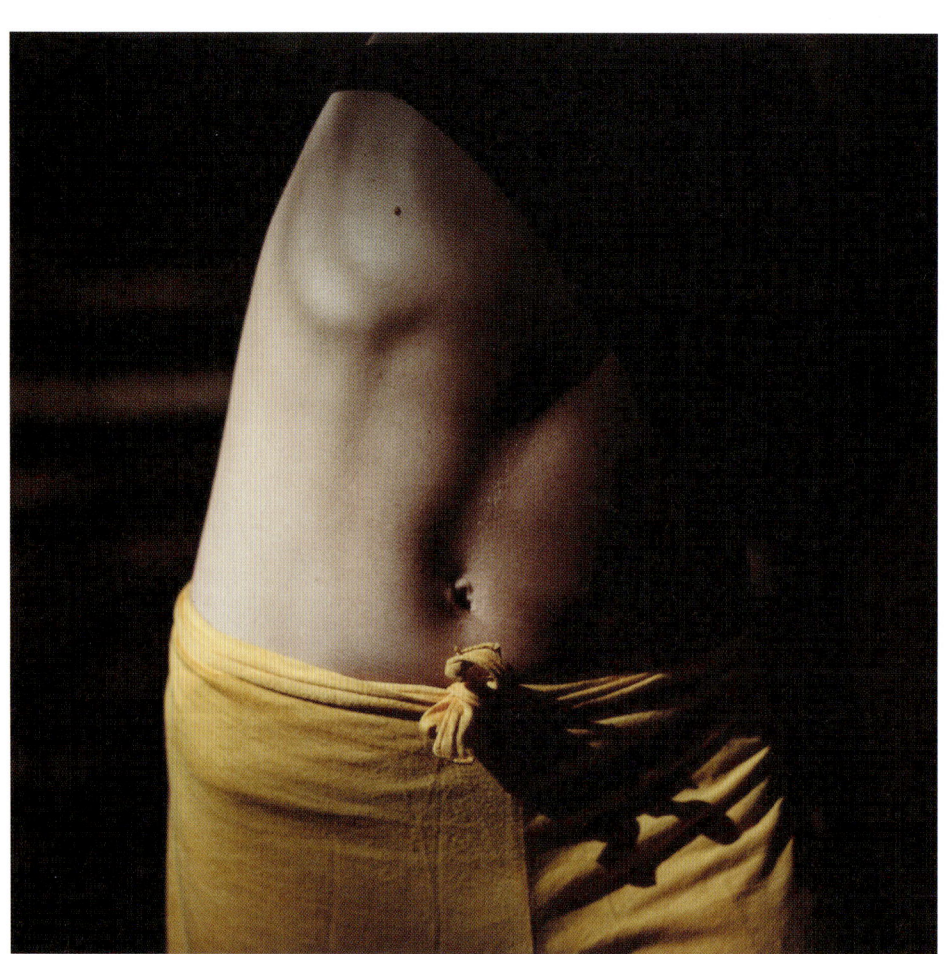

7

MINDS AND HEARTS

The feeling is evident. As we loosen our hold we sense from the heart. For centuries spiritual teachers have pointed to altruistic love, an experience of compassion, warm enveloping friendliness, a shared awakening, peace, tenderness, empathy, and deep unitive awareness.

Such experiences are valuable if only to remind us they are not easily sustained. We may take the unified experience into life but habitual patterns get in the way. *Deciding* to love can be fruitful when based on group experiences. Without the mind to tell us we love, we would not know that we loved, but the mind can interfere with love. Minds are dominated by thought, not love. We cannot think ourselves into love or summon love on demand. Thinking into love needs the support of feeling good for love of the whole to manifest. The ego recognizes love but does not produce it. The ego cannot love *just like that*. Reducing the grip of the ego, softening its presence, encourages loving feelings. Altruistic love can spring undeterred from a spontaneous adjustment of the mind that softens rational consciousness. Love is involuntary.

Love is complex because we are complex. Maternal, familial, platonic, romantic, and erotic love are common ground and may be enduring, fleeting, transitory, or unpredictable. Exclusive love fosters possessive behavior, while love of the whole is free from attachment. Unconditional love is free from an object of love, although love for someone can exist in tandem with love of the whole. Loving a person can be complicated by conditioning and may benefit from a universal perspective. The unitive love arising in group work feels like a religious experience as we reconnect. The word *religion* comes from the Latin *religiere* meaning *to connect again*.

There are numerous books on love's nature, its values, and how to love. We know love's importance, can study its chemistry, and are aware that the science of love pales in the wake of the feeling. The philosophy of love reminds us of love but cannot instill the experience. Warm, empathetic, loving friendliness arises spontaneously from the body and registers in subliminal consciousness, the mind, and the softening ego. Love is sublime. It spreads outward, a quiet, connective, sensitive awareness to the feelings

Chapter 7

of others. I have rarely, if ever, left a class without that shared feeling having arisen. When the mind empties, we approach one another without need.

Self-love

A group experiencing love is made up of individuals experiencing *their* love. Personal love feeds and in turn is fed by the group. It begins with how we treat ourselves. As we have heard many times, we might begin by remembering to love ourselves. Loving ourselves (a little) more opens a door. Approaching ourselves with calm interest, sincerity, patience, and kindness opens our hearts, enabling us to extend these qualities to others. It begins by giving ourselves *time* to open, get out of our own way and enable the onset of pleasurable expansion. Self-kindness involves self-acknowledgment, self-appreciation, self-awareness, self-acceptance, and a measure of quiet self-adjustment.

Conditioning affects us deeply. The gurus and spiritual guides understood through their own experience that no one has ideal internal behavior. A feeling of self-forgiveness can arise in group work. We might not know what we forgive ourselves for (being us). It is a feeling that arises from ego release and dissolving the tension of self-expectation. Forgiveness is a sense. We can notice our behavior and be kind to what we notice. The extraordinary thing is that *softly noticing* changes behavior effortlessly and immediately.

A self-caring attitude provides a basis for empathetic behavior. Self-noticing deepens and broadens the scope of teaching. The quality of our emotional experience, our interest in the experience of others, and how they may be feeling is the foundation for group cohesion. Unmitigated self-kindness fosters calmness, informs language, the timing of words, and the pace of the work. As things get underway, self-kindness occupies the background of awareness but may come to the foreground when we find ourselves in territory needing more sensitivity. Self-caring awareness, free from *thinking about* self-caring, enhances expansion and confidence, softens group texture, and provides fertile soil for the emergence of compassionate energy. When the mind is quietly attentive to itself the heart opens. For some, love may lie just beneath the surface, a breath or two away; for others, it may hide within patterns from the past. Change takes the time it needs. Trust comes from self-kindness. If altruistic love begins within one's own heart, it must pass through one's own self to reach others.

> Lying on your back, with your arms open, let your awareness hover gently above and then touch the skin covering your breast bone. Delicately pass through the tissues. With infinite lightness, move around your heart. Feel space between your breastbone and heart, between your heart and the floor, and between your heart and elbows. Feel your heart dissolve and radiate into the space around you. Take the group into the experience with you. Unvarnished love dissolves thought and the absence of thought reveals love.

Minds and hearts

Love and thought

How can the thinking mind impede love? The possibility that thought can inhibit love may seem unlikely to those unfamiliar with mysticism or yoga and even to some who are. I love my child and thought cannot deter my love. Thinking about those I love can fill me with love, although such thoughts may contain an element of ambiguity. But quiet, unattached, unitive love is impeded by thought because thought is conditioned. Thought, built on conditioned experience acts as a screen between oneself and unitive, unsentimental love. We might think and love simultaneously, but it is a matter of intensity. The yogic slant on love is a blissful experience that relinquishes thought at the time of the experience. The transience of unitive love appears inevitable. We can take it as it comes while opting for the promise of a more enduring possibility.

Enlightened obstetrician Michel Odent observed that the intensity of loving feelings during birth is reduced by stimulating the intellect. Conversely a reduction in neocortical activity (thought) enhances unitive love, a common experience during and following birth (Odent 1999). We feel love emerge during expansive sensations and may be aware of the line between enhancing or disturbing the involuntary process of love. The intellect disturbs the natural flow of loving feelings, but the mind's acknowledgment of love can enhance it. Altruistic love flourishes when thought and analysis are at the periphery of awareness.

We are conditioned to think that our thinking is us. What and how we think is an essential signature of individuality. But thought is not the whole of us; yet thinking cannot turn itself off, and when it does it returns in a moment to tell itself it is turned off by which time it is too late! Unconditioned love, for the time that it lasts, cannot survive

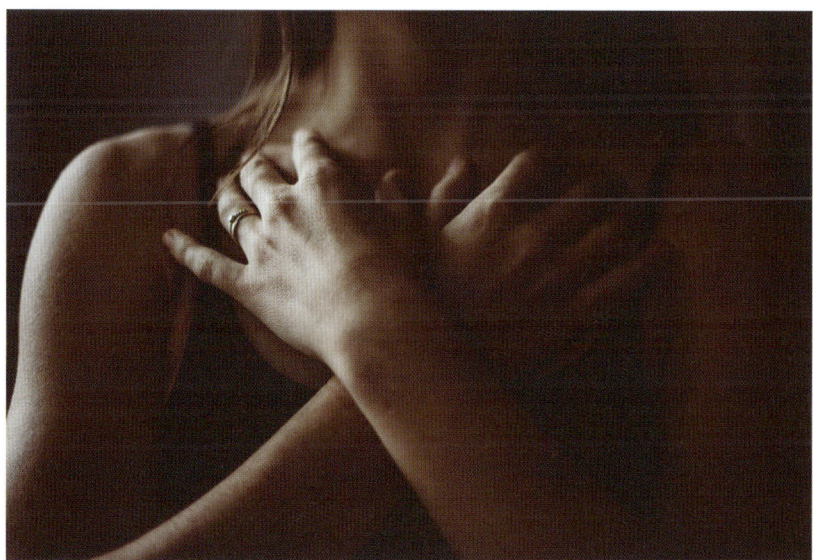

When the mind is quietly attentive to itself the heart opens. For some, love may lie just beneath the surface, a breath away; for others, love may hide within patterns of the past.

a mind disturbed by the fragmentary nature of thought.

The mind continually disturbs itself by thought, which is a fragment of consciousness. The practice of unthinking is recommended by the more radical spiritual teachers. This takes a step further than standing aside and witnessing thought pass by without attachment. The absence of thought has more impact than observing the movement of thought. Thought is a barrier between oneself and altruistic love in its purest form. Unthinking is an unusual experience, interrupted by the mind's opportunistic compulsion to describe the experience of not thinking.

> A useful experiment is to love your thinking! You will notice that thought disappears as you love it. Thought cannot handle love. Thought is overwhelmed by love, and the sensation of love is more powerful than thought! If you can love yourself you can love your thinking and you will notice that thought yields to love. If you go into what kind of love loving your thinking is you will see it is simply calm and caring noticing.

Awakening depth awakens a love that is impeded by stimulating the intellect. Sensation is a realistic alternative to thought. Thinking yields to the more ancient phenomenon of loving sensations. Quiet, expansive, all-encompassing sensations draw out our love. Love proliferates when thought is in the background. We know from experience that the quality of our teaching is optimized when the intellect is quiet.

Mystic love

Mystical experience feels like love. Mystical experiences manifest through shifts in consciousness. Deeper consciousness invites mystic love. Mystics observe their minds as a practice and a way of being. The words mystic, mysticism, and mystery come from the Latin *mystes*. Mystic is defined as *occult* or *secret,* and *mystical* is defined as *enigmatic, obscure, symbolic,* or *having a spiritual significance or value*. Mysticism implies an interest in the mysterious. The attraction of the mysterious is found in its unlimited space and vastness. Mysticism seeks freedom in the unknown. We cannot examine the unknown, because it is unknowable, but we can consider its presence and ponder its meaning. Should the unknown become known it would lose its value. Accepting an unknown contributes to the depth and quality of our work. Mystic love is love of the unknown, a love of nothing in particular, and a love of something larger than ourselves. Love of the unknown releases feelings of unitive love. The feeling of something infinite draws out our personal capacity to love. Group work enhances sensations that promote *aha* moments and lays the foundation for spiritual experience and insight. Should a universal love exist, it would express itself through us, and we oblige by clearing the way, by removing patterns that inhibit loving feelings.

Working on our selves, in the company of others working on their selves, has unknown undertones. *We do not know where it is going*. A mystical element prevails. Mysticism is as much a feeling of possibility as anything else and can be seen as a spiritual emotion. Perhaps the unknown

Minds and hearts

fosters love because it lacks an object that might breed possessiveness, ambiguity, or disillusionment. Mystic experiences indicate we have transcended knowledge, ideas, and habitual thought.

The ego provides the viewpoint from which we can see love from a personal perspective. Ancient aspects of consciousness provide the feeling of expansive unity.

Attention is love

Being attentive is an act of love because attention reflects an interest in relationship. Whether attention moves inward toward ourselves or outward to others it has the same quality. Attention and love have contributed to our evolutionary continuance. Attention is an indication of love, and love comes to our attention. Attention, love, and consciousness are woven from the same evolutionary cloth.

Focused attention and a deepening consciousness lead to more love. Total attention requires the absence of superfluous activity and necessitates being in the moment. Factors that inhibit love are loosened when we are in the present. References to the past or future, ideas on what just happened or should happen, sully the flow of the undisturbed attention that promotes love.

Attention is initially an act of will until it becomes spontaneous. Love is not an act of will. Love is involuntary. The will is influenced by conditioning and therefore unreliable as a tool for entering into the expansive emotion of love. Love arises from quiet and sustained attention. Attention changes the texture of relationship and is felt by those we are attentive to and attentive with. Group attention promotes group love.

> As your rational mind lifts and the quality of your attention deepens, notice how going into yourself with kindness unfolds into a unitive attentiveness toward the group and everyone in it. You express spatial love that takes in all within your field of awareness. It touches the group, and they return it in kind.

Love is sensation

Every emotional nuance has a physical basis, some register in awareness and some do not. A host of physical sensations accompany ever-changing emotional activity. All categories of love are rooted in the body as physical experiences. Love, along with its nemesis fear, is a primary emotion felt by the body and registered in the sensory mind. According to William James emotions generally are "emotional brain-processes [that] not only resemble the ordinary sensorial brain-processes, but in very truth are nothing but such processes variously combined" (James 1884).

It is accepted and often experienced that the mental perception of something creates an emotion that gives rise to physical changes. It is also accepted that the physical changes are the emotion. Emotions vary between strong or weak sensations. Sensation has emotional

Chapter 7

content and emotions are recognized by their sensations. Sensation and emotion share a theatre of awareness. The sensation of touching someone for the first time can have a powerful emotional resonance. Physical expression invokes emotion.

The involuntary expansion of the body and consciously allowing the body to open can have profound emotional content. Opening the skin of the legs and shoulders arouses the emotion of freedom. Opening the skin over the heart induces the emotion of love and/or vulnerability.

The yogi attempted to transcend emotion by transcending sensation and free himself from emotionally driven activity. He directed consciousness into his sensory emotional experience in order to dissolve it. For him, consciousness was larger and more penetrative than its content. He endeavoured to transcend emotion in order to be unaffected by life. If we are *in* life, it is impossible not to be affected *by* life, and on some level we would not wish to be unaffected by life. Altruistic love, one of our greatest gifts, can be courted, celebrated, and where possible introduced into life. The sensation of love is a regular experience in groups because we continually revert to pleasant sensations.

Expansion is love

Expansion and contraction are primary expressions of emotive life. Expansion is an expression of pleasure, and contraction is an expression of displeasure. Expansive and contractive moods compete for predominance.

French philosopher Alfred Fouillée wrote:

The movement of concentration upon self and of the defensive [attitude], common to all personal or egotistical feelings, gives to their expression ... a character essentially concentric or centripetal, while the expression of the benevolent affections is centrifugal and "eccentric." Fear presents the type of the concentric physiognomy pertaining to the affections which have for their center the me. ... it is the correlative movement of organic expansion or contraction that is the real generator of the language of the emotions. (Fouillée 1887)

Expansion is a joyful and spiritually emotive expression. The more expansive we are the more profound the experience of love. The degree of expansion is proportional to the intensity of the feeling. The altruistic feeling of goodwill is an expansive emotion that predominates when contractive emotion dissolves. Love is expansive and expansion invites love. The feeling of love may inspire us to use the *word* love with those we are in expansion with and when the timing feels right. The word love has an ambiguous connotation, reminding us that we may not love. The words (be) *amazed* and (feel) *wonder* are connected to expansive loving feelings and easy to use. They well up spontaneously when we are in amazement and *wondrous*.

MINDS AND HEARTS

> Now, as you read, go into expansion – not as an exercise but simply imagine yourself expanding and radiating through your skin in all directions. Emote outward. You may notice it is hard to have distinct thoughts as you expand. Expansion dissolves intrusive thought and invites more love. It is amazing!

Expansion is a sensory emotional experience radiating outward from a center. Love comes when we move out from ourselves. We remain present (self-kindness) but are less *self*-centered. Expansionary consciousness touches the surrounding space and the group connects with emotional oneness. Kindness and spatial sensations emote as one feeling. We flow outward giving ourselves away from a clear and soft sense of self. Unitive love is nonpossessive and inclusive. Physical, emotional, and mental space promote loving feelings that emerge through a dissolving screen of conditioning. "The fact is that the mystical feeling of enlargement, union, and emancipation has no specific intellectual content whatever of its own" (James 1902/2018).

Emotive consciousness

As the mind empties and its content reduces, the inner space of consciousness can feel vast, as if sealed from external interference, with the odd thought or registration seeping through. Unmitigated consciousness is a radiation that starts with a feeling of inner space and, like an emotion, emanates into surrounding space. Antonio Damasio's proposal that emotion and attention have been implicit in the development of consciousness supports the experience of consciousness as an emotive force (Damasio 2000). At some point during the process consciousness becomes *the* primary emotion. A pure or superconsciousness can be seen as the condition of love but without the familiar emotionality, simply aware of its own presence, devoid of object or content. During deep and expansive group work the emotion of consciousness takes over as the patchwork of well-known emotions recede. The *one with everything* feeling could touch on a core self or an archaic consciousness. We may awaken a way of being that was the norm before neocortical control gained ascendance. Freud felt that: "The unconscious drive is not only instinctual, but also the Eros of the personal unconscious, augmented by creativity from the collective unconscious" (Freud 1927/1962). In other words as our personal and group unconscious surfaces, it is accompanied by emergent love.

Sensations register in the sensory cortex, an area intimately tied to the neocortex, the thinking or rational brain. Emotional feeling and mental activity are inseparable. We know, or should know, how we feel. We are generally, but not always, conscious of our feelings. Awareness and consciousness can be seen as primary emotions that highlight and penetrate the emotional flux that rolls by, on a more or less continual basis.

Newborn babies have an undeveloped neocortex and lack a sense of self (Odent 1999). Archaic and magical consciousness preceded individuality. Our sense of being separate is born out of an original sense of "oneness" that we return to as we transcend our selves.

Chapter 7

Such occasions underpin our potential for profound insight and invite a language, tone, and timing that opens the experience to the group. The natural, undisturbed movement of pure dynamic consciousness can feel like love set free as we let go of the experience of love.

Love and conditioning

Unconditioned love is not necessarily unconditional love (love free from conditions). Unconditioned love is a lucid awareness of the presence of a love not conditioned by experiences or filtered through a screen of conditioning. Love strengthens as conditioning drops away. Unitive love comes more easily to some than others. Conditioned minds coexist with conditioned hearts. Fixed ideas may limit the scope of love. A closed heart may limit the scope of the mind and a conditioned mind may limit the scope of the heart. Conditioning strengthens selfish needs.

Softening our *selves* invites a unitive heart and mind. An all-encompassing expansion arises with unconditioned love. Awareness enables the acknowledgment of love's presence. Archaic and magical man may have felt a unitive love due to the absence of rational consciousness. When free to roam, unitive love runs parallel with a sense of wonder.

Intimacy

Intimacy comes from the Latin word *intima* meaning *innermost*. A field of intimacy can be felt as our innermost selves release profound energy. There is a feeling of merging with one another like one organism opening and transforming. We become intimate with those around us, with the surrounding space touching our skin, and with the radiation of inner space. A *knowing* contains and spreads an ongoing sense of oneness. Group love is enhanced by accepting the consciousness of others. Love is found where consciousnesses meet. The consciousness of all penetrates and transforms internal behavior. The more we go into and beyond our selves the more intimate we feel. Intimacy assuages shyness, dissolves barriers, gives a deep sense of connection to oneself and others, and invites love.

The essential aspect of our immediate environment is one another, a realization amplified in groups. We deeply connect as we drop beneath separative veneers of habit. Superficiality, the social tool serving daily communication, is blown away by the depth of the process at hand as we share the intensification of an empathetic field. Observations and insights may or may not include the love word. Its reality is in the room, like a bright and gentle mist. The mind knows love through feelings made conscious. Cultivating mental space invites the proliferation of loving kindness. Alfred Fouillée observed:

The instinctive reaction of the will under the influence of the feeling, having been extended by contagion to similar organisms, and, if other men comprehend what we feel, it is because they themselves feel it. The final result of this sympathetic communication is the retranslation of the emotion felt by one into similar emotions in the others. The emotion of our neighbor is returned to us by a kind of response …

Minds and hearts

Seeing the movements and attitudes of others we tend to realize them in ourselves; then, as by a counter-stroke, the movement and attitude by us to reproduce in us the feelings that correspond to them.
(Fouillée 1887)

Some facts of unconditioned love

- The sensory mind is more in touch with love than the thinking mind

- Thought is ambiguous, and it impedes unconditioned love

- Unconditioned love is unambiguous

- Thought strengthens thought, and love strengthens love

- The mind may inhibit or enhance love

- Love tempers the mind

- The ultimate freedom is in loving

- Spatial consciousness radiates love.

Limbic love

The triune brain theory, one that modern science dismisses as simplistic, sheds a little light on love. The theory proposes that our brain is made up of three brains. Our behavior has evolved out of the successive evolution of three anatomical structures, and from the bottom to the top these are:

- *An ancient reptilian brain*, represented by the expanded continuation of the spinal cord, is responsible for controlling and regulating vital functions such as respiration and heart pulsation. The reptilian brain is devoid of mammalian characteristics and cannot produce emotion. Cold-blooded reptiles do not love (as far as we can tell).

- *A limbic brain* (from the Latin word *limbus* meaning *border*) differentiates the reptilian from the mammalian brain, mammalian life being the next evolutionary stage toward human development. Early mammals showed the first signs of taking care of their offspring and bonding in groups. The limbic brain is said to be responsible for emotional life.

- *A neocortical brain,* the largest more recent brain, is apparently still expanding, as its numerous functions, still not fully understood, continue to evolve. The limbic brain produces the emotions that direct the cortical brain and stimulate the thoughts and appropriate action for any given scenario.

The *limbic* brain continually converts sensory data into emotional activity, a fact that highlights the relationship between sensation and love. The *limbic* brain, also known as the *limbic* system, is concerned with bonding, human relationships, and the survival of the species by installing appropriate caring strategies. Love (and other emotions) arises from the limbic system to be processed by the sensory and thinking cortex. When we are stimulated by sensations (of love),

Chapter 7

we find expression through the language of the cortex and guide others accordingly. The inspired book *A General Theory of Love* proposes "the entire neo-cortex is driven by the paralimbic regions from which it evolved … 'Rhythmic wording' appears to link the limbic and neocortical area of the brain" (Lewis et al. 2000). If we wonder how we find the intonations and rhythm to convey sensation and make effective suggestions this may provide an answer.

Our ability to sense emotion in others arises from the limbic brain. "Emotionality is the social sense organ of limbic creatures … emotionality enables a mammal to sense the inner states and the motives of the mammals around him." Our ability to adapt our emotions to the emotions of others is described as "limbic resonance." "A mammal can detect the internal state of another mammal and adjust its own physiology to match the situation – a change in turn sensed by the other, who likewise adjusts. … a symphony of mutual exchange and internal adaption whereby two mammals become attuned to each other's inner states" (Lewis et al. 2000).

Limbic resonance pervades groups and harmonizes the transition between habitual patterns and profound transformation. Sharing space with others for hours or days at a time, with a common focus on attention, awareness, and sensation, stimulates limbic ways of being. Sensing together, we become more aware of one another's emotions. Coexperiencing, we peer into our collective depth. "… limbic states can leap between minds, feelings are contagious" (Lewis et al. 2000). The yogi penetrated his mind, entered the far reaches of consciousness and the deep limbic areas of his brain, but without knowing it in that way.

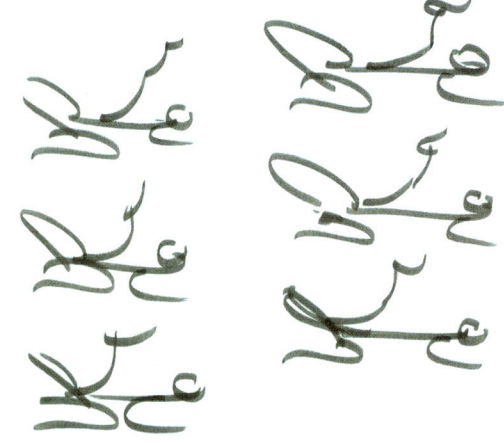

Limbic states can leap between minds. Feelings are contagious.

The chemistry of unconditioned love

We are told that love creates significant changes in blood chemistry. Lewis et al. (2000) point out that the neural pathways for emotion and intellect are separate. But the chemical relationship between the heart and mind is unquestionable. The brain and heart act as glands that secrete oxytocin, the hormone of love. The chemistry of love diffuses throughout the entire system.

The physiology of love lies beyond the limbic system. Receptors all over the body are sensitive to oxytocin. They are richly distributed in the female reproductive system and are found in the heart, the primitive brain, the vascular system, and the digestive and immune systems. Research suggests that more and more sites are found to be sensitive to, and release, oxytocin. Pleasurable expansion releases oxytocin, the hormone of kindness, love, and calmness. Living tissue responds to oxytocin and stimulates its release. The tissues love!

A chemistry of expansion would involve oxytocin release and ascendance, while a chemistry of contraction or resistance would involve adrenalin predominance. Engaging with excessive resistance can provoke an initial adrenal response. Giving time for expansion, from an attitude of kindness and care, would release an oxytocin predominance from the beginning. We lack the means to read the chemistry but we have the direct experience. Surface tissue is rich in oxytocin receptors and this would explain the pleasurable sensations arising from expansion, should we need the confirmation.

Thought would have a similar chemistry. Loving, gentle thought would be oxytocin based, while ambitious or even expectant thought might foster adrenalin release. Kind thoughts release the chemistry of kindness. We cannot will our mind to empty, but the chemistry of kindness might be a route to the chemistry of emptiness. Unitive love arises when the mind is empty. The absence of thought and the presence of expansion share the same chemistry.

The point is that, when activated, the glandular nature of the brain tends to reduce neocortical activity, as shown in studies on childbirth (Odent 1999). The absence of thought produces loving feelings, and, in turn, loving feelings reduce thought. All-inclusive feelings of love are diffuse and include love of one's self, gently swept up in love of the whole. We love love itself.

Oxytocin released into the brain influences our behavior, dissolves anxiety, and makes us feel like bonding. Oxytocin is the hormone of connectivity, fostering trust and a deeper sense of vastness. Research shows that oxytocin enables us to assess other people's emotions, an essential factor in holding and guiding groups. Oxytocin softens heart tissue, and this can be felt and suggested to others. Being present with your heart, giving it quiet attention, visualizing and sensing space around and within your heart, releases oxytocin and reduces thought.

If oxytocin is the hormone of love, it is also the hormone of transcendence. Oxytocin release is enhanced many times in a group transcending their conditioning. People remark how group chemistry works so well. The observation is literal. People connect and release oxytocin. Groups bond through pleasurable sensations.

Alexander Lowen observed: "On the unconscious level all activities are instinctual, all impulses are equal and unitary, and all can be reduced to the common principle: the pleasure principle" (Lowen 1958). At the most basic level we need and seek pleasure. This need, and its resolution, is made conscious as we strip away the impediments of conditioned behavior.

A little science is useful. The science of love is not love itself and does not guarantee the experience of love. Knowing the limbic brain is the mammalian center of love does not produce love. Thinking of oxytocin or limbic activity does not enhance love and may even inhibit it. The intellectualization of feeling veils the feeling. Referring to love's chemistry

Chapter 7

and our mammalian origins shows that we know our stuff. Alongside the actual experience, many students are encouraged by this kind of information. There is probably research in the making that deepens the objective understanding of altruistic love and behavior, but knowledge cannot replace the skill needed to reveal and sustain love. There may be a resistance to the details that attempt to prove the existence of something so natural, joyful, and fulfilling as love. Students are open to supportive information, but opening the heart and keeping it open is the key to loving ourselves and each other a little more.

We do not measure oxytocin release or limbic activity in class work, but we do bathe together in love's light. Love is assisted by acknowledging the emotional texture of relationship.

Vulnerability

Opening hearts reveals vulnerability. Students may at first feel vulnerable as defences come down. Some may mask vulnerability while others have no need. Vulnerability arises as the familiarity of the ego disperses. Allowing, and being with vulnerability is an aspect of spiritual wisdom. In this sense vulnerability does not imply feeling weak or unable to cope, but implies a soft, adaptive exposure, an unguarded transparency, as all experience passes through consciousness and through the body. We should defend ourselves through choice but not habit. We can respond with a soft mind, a gentle tone, without losing our sense of purpose. Saying no with undisturbed, undefended composure is surprisingly effective. An undefended self has an inner strength that connects with others, merges with surrounding fields, and receives and transmits ways of being, with or without the spoken word.

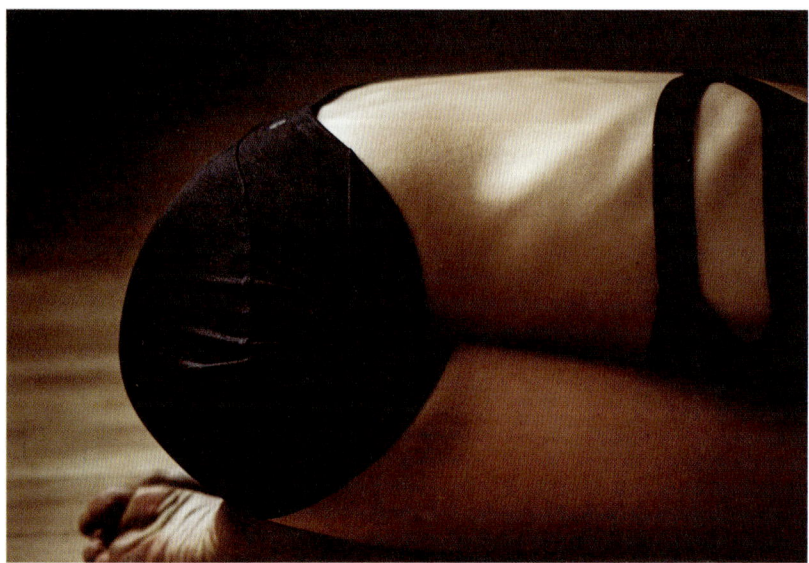

An undefended self has an inner strength that connects with others, merges with surrounding fields, and receives and transmits ways of being, with or without the spoken word.

Minds and hearts

> When deeply engaged with a group, be vulnerable. We may speak and act in ways that are subtly defensive. Proving ourselves as teachers may feel necessary at times but inhibits deeper communication. Feel space over your heart, feel outside space gently enter your inner heart space, and sense your heart soften, lighten, and dissolve to become part of the space surrounding it and you. Draw attention to vulnerability while feeling vulnerable. Remain open and allow pure consciousness to emerge. You may begin to smile!

A strong sense of self is undefended and trusts. Vulnerability requires self-trust and may take a little courage. As mentioned, the word "courage" comes from the old French *corage* which means heart. A courageous heart is present, open, generous, calm, responsive, and unaffected by what happens. In this respect vulnerability is invulnerability. We are already vulnerable. There is nowhere to go from there, nothing to defend. Courage exists at the heart of love.

Prayer and privacy

Groups commune. Expanding together feels like prayer. We "pray" to and from the best part of ourselves and one another. We pray *through* ourselves, to a love of the whole. Obstetrician Michel Odent noticed women in labor at some point needed to be unobserved. If there were others present a woman would adopt a forward-bending attitude. To avoid the gaze of others she would bend over something or go on all fours, an attitude not only mechanically advantageous for labor but one indicating a need for privacy, much like praying (Odent 1999).

Bending forward has significant implications. The privacy afforded by bending forward enables us to access a deeper process. We can spend longer in these attitudes while engaging with the sensation of expansion. We may not register a praying experience, but the feeling it gives is one of praying to a unitive state. Nonexposure, the fact of not being seen, enhances the emergence of subliminal consciousness. As the private experience deepens, the love field of the group intensifies. Active communion acknowledges spatial consciousness as a temple of worship. Personal and group consciousness blends to produce a state of grace.

> From an easy sitting, forward-bending position, add a quiet intimacy to the tone of your voice. As expansion takes over and the field thickens, refer to the nature of prayer.

The inner Buddhist

We have an inner Buddhist. William James's suggestion that Buddhism was pessimistic may have been due to its philosophy that life was suffering. But Buddhism advocates compassion and joy for the very reason people suffer, many without knowing it. Buddhism revolves around a realization that we may all know at heart. Compassion is an emotion that arises from gentle detachment. We may, in principle, be familiar with the middle path even if we do not always tread it. Being pulled this way or that takes up

Chapter 7

the foreground unless we learn to notice. Milarepa the Buddhist sage had this to say:

The nature of Mind is Emptiness and Luminosity
Inseparably conjoined …
Spontaneously merging with that original state
I am indifferent to experiences of good and bad

With mind free and effortless, I rest in happiness and joy.
Where subject and object are realized as a single sphere
Happiness and sorrow mingle as one …
Whatever circumstances I encounter
I am free in the blissful realm of self-awakening Wisdom. (Baker 2004)

The Tibetan word *sem* has an all-encompassing meaning. It takes in heart, mind, and spirit. Tibetan Buddhists see no difference between these three. The heart is the integral part of all aspects of ourselves. The underlying philosophy of Buddha-nature suggests that compassion is inherent but is buried by negative conditioning built up by a dominance of the selfish aspects of the ego. Beneath this we are naturally benevolent.

Altruistic behavior is conducive to the survival of the species. Caring for one another in groups supports the group's continuance. Studies also show that the most self-focused people, those that continually use "I" and "me" in conversation and lack close social relationships, were more prone to heart disease, unhappiness, and more vulnerable to ill health generally (The Dalai Lama & Cutler 1998). Group work that invites the love field has far-reaching effects.

It is necessary to understand the mind and heart in relationships. Does the heart have a mind? Is there any heart in the mind? Tibetan Buddhists put their hand on their heart when they refer to the mind. We may be unaware of our inner Buddhist but a practicing *person* might suffice. If or when we seek spiritual understanding, we might simply accept the love inside us.

Quantum love

Emotions can be seen as tides of energy within a larger field. Love's neurochemistry and love's experience may break down into quantum and morphic fields that spread out indefinitely. We may bond through emotional interactions that move out from personal centers via quantum and morphic resonance, passing through the connective tissue of space. A quantum messenger carries love between us. Quantum physics defies separation: there are no *things*, simply a unified interconnecting fabric. Organic matter and space are continuous but exist as different densities. We are condensations of space and space is the decondensation of us. Love's spread, devoid of object, may, unsentimentally and without attachment, weave its way through the fabric of existence. In passing through us, quantum love may condense to become an emotion to be felt and expressed, hence the Eastern proposal that life's purpose is to express universal love.

The powerful nonpossessive sense of belonging to the whole and to one another may be love's intention. A group can be experienced as one organism, inseparable from and resonating with a grand design. If, as teachers, we recognize a larger experience due to the sensitivity between our hearts, minds, and bodies, we cannot help but offer these possibilities to others. The way to the heart is from the heart and includes space and self-surrendering made conscious to the group.

Choosing love

We can choose love, as it passes. If love chooses us, we might share it. A stable sense of self supporting the vulnerability of love speaks for itself. We do not distribute love but acknowledge its presence. It can take time for some students to accept themselves; for others, it takes no time at all. When we slow right down, we can draw attention to love's transience. The mind can choose and the heart follows. Positive emotion can endure for longer periods.

For most of us a love of the whole does not last in its purest form. Freud commented that not everyone was worthy of love, which is a bleak view. Freud was not a spiritual teacher, nor did he profess to be one. Others, more spiritually oriented, would say that love can be found in everyone. We change as impeding factors drop away. Heightened awareness may be a subtle expression of love's presence. Those feeling unworthy of love may be carried by the flow. We may not need the words love or compassion. The reality is a calm tenderness, a patient attitude, and an empathetic strategy. Choosing to accept loving feelings leads toward love's choiceless state.

The smallest shift

Significant light bulb moments, although transcendently welcome, may not be a frequent occurrence. Change can involve a lighter touch. Love amongst groups can involve the smallest shift. Five or ten percent more love permeates body and soul and ignites the probability of more love. Understanding this dissolves the impossibility of "I should love more." The propensity is there beneath the surface and may be immediate. The mind remembers love, and consciousness embraces it. Perhaps the neocortex, the limbic system, and the tissues acknowledge one another's presence. Remembering acts as a switch, we can turn the light on.

> Give love the time it needs to show itself. Love emerges as expectation evaporates. There is love in satisfaction and satisfaction in love. Let it be enough!

I have yet to meet a spiritual teacher who, having focused on awakening his consciousness, does not have an open heart, or, having focused on opening his heart, does not have an awakened consciousness.

Universal love may be beyond altruistic love while also including it! When consciousness is totally clear, when we move between attention to and awareness of a purer consciousness, we reveal an unsentimental, serene, all-encompassing yet penetrant energy that feels as if it touches the nature of existence. We might not recognize this feeling as love, but it might be love in its essential form, a love not sullied by our recognition.

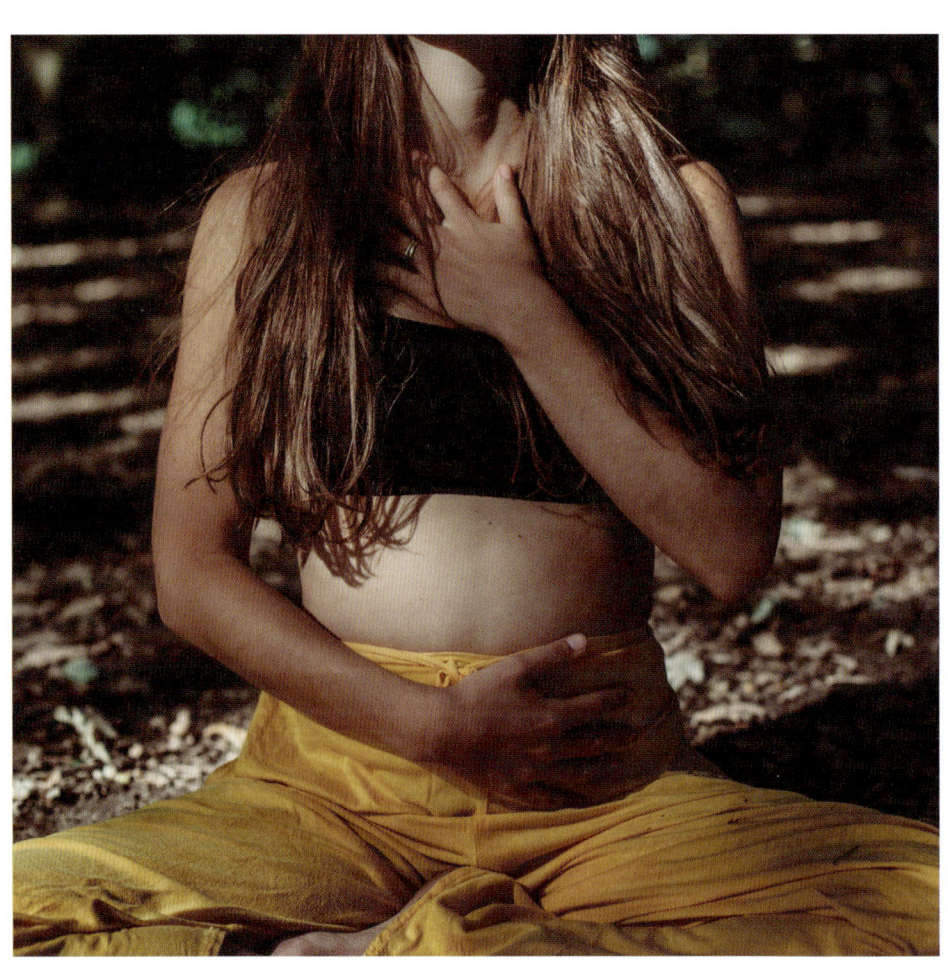

Insight and wisdom 8

Insight wells up as conditioning dissolves, making a profound contribution to group experience.

We light up as insights surface. Insight accompanies heightened sensation, meaningful silence, and space. The understanding that a guru speaks from his own experience, that he knows the emotional pulls, and is personally acquainted with turbulence and conflict is the first insight. Realizing that we all have personal alternatives is also an insight. Insights are enlightened realizations or feelings that emote, and they move out from within, expressed as an understanding or "seeing." Insights are spontaneous teaching tools highlighting the reality of the moment. We cannot teach others *how* to have insight, but we can open a field of realization by expressing our own insights. Once expressed, the feeling and the space remains for the insightfulness of others to flourish.

The understanding that emptiness is a precondition for insight, that our bodies are inseparable from space, that we are all conditioned, and that insightfulness is a creative aspect of our work are primary insights based on fact.

Insights surface:

- in tandem with enlightened physical sensation

- when patterns of conditioning soften

- from a deeper body experience

- when thought is absent or in the background of awareness

- when rational consciousness has emptied

- when we *know* without content

- when we accept the nature of space

- when awakened lucidity prevails.

Insights surface again and again and, although expressed through personal interpretation, refer to the same theme,

Chapter 8

namely what lies beneath or beyond our conditioned minds, for example:

- Undisturbed awareness is a movement. It flows.

- Perception is immediate action.

- A strong sense of self has no center. It comes from pure observation.

- Space is the ultimate center.

- Emotions control behavior and impede lucid awakening.

- Observing emotion dissolves attachment.

- Unconditioned observation is choiceless.

- Insight frees us from past experience (at the time).

- Thought is based on the accumulation of experience.

- The rational mind has a tendency to be irrational.

- We may have an idea to go from here to there, but we are already there. By moving toward there we lose what is here.

- It does not matter – it is just an experience.

- There is an extraordinary depth to being present.

- We are trapped by projections, expectations, and wants.

- Everything arrives when we stop looking.

- Consciousness is most dynamic when free from content.

- Conscience is the defining factor of human consciousness, our compass. Without conscience there is no point.

- Love is the ultimate wisdom.

Coming to mind

Insight emerges when we release conditioned patterns of tension. A proliferation of insight may follow the release of energy that binds these patterns. A reservoir of wisdom surfaces as personal realizations are shared in our own language. Insights are inspired condensations of the *state* of wisdom. The Shorter Oxford English dictionary defines *insight* as *"internal sight; mental vision or perception; a glimpse or view beneath the surface."*

The source of insight might lie in archaic, magical, or mythical consciousness. The energy driving insight might spring from Damasio's core self or Freud's preconscious to combine with current fields of understanding. The unknown origin of insight adds to its potency and appeals to our inner mystic. Quotes from past authorities inspire but lack the potency of on-the-spot experiential

Insight and wisdom

insight arriving into clear and present consciousness. William James could be right in his belief that universal consciousness is simply the exposure of subliminal consciousness. On the other hand, it may be that subliminal consciousness has to download universal consciousness. The art is in delivering *aha* moments, regardless of the source.

Penetrant insight

There is no such thing as a shallow insight because insight arises from beneath or beyond rational consciousness. Insight highlights a deeper reality, is spiritual in nature, and invokes a higher creativity. Penetrant insight moves us beyond ongoing experience and releases inspired realizations from a deep and broad field of consciousness.

How insights arise is no clearer than how a mind or consciousness arises. Beyond the conditions that release insights, it is unknown how they are given wings. It is clear, however, that profound insight occurs when (and to whatever degree or for however long) conditioning is suspended. Suspension implies a cessation of activity that impedes flowing outness. Impeding activity may be as subtle as a slight intention or expectation.

The physicist David Bohm commented:

the suggestion is that insight is an intelligence beyond any of the energies that could be defined in thought. ... It's the insight not you. ... the insight being supreme intelligence is able to rearrange the very structural matter of the brain which underlies thought ... leaving the brain open to perceive reality in a different way. **(Bohm in Wilber 1982)**

> As awareness moves through, around, and beyond your body, observe how insight follows expansive sensations. Tissue intelligence stimulates realization.

Prescience, instinct, and intuition

The word *prescience* means *to know before*, from the Latin *pre* meaning *before* and *scire* meaning *to know*. When we are *prescient* our sense of *knowing* is woven into consciousness. Insight is based on a prescient awakening crystallized into thought words by the ego. Philosophical and spiritual insight is linked to instinct and intuition. Instinct is based on a primal sense whereas intuition gives us a conscious feeling *about* something. Intuition goes beyond instinct. We *have* instinct and we *intuit*. Both arise from beneath rational consciousness and are rooted in the body. We have a *feeling* about something. The tissues feel the imminence of insight; they *know* just before an insight is released into consciousness. A wave of insightful consciousness passes through the body as a sensation.

Philosopher Henri Bergson believed that human intuition is founded on the instinct of animals "like a painter's capacity for pure perception it [instinct] apprehends the world directly, yielding knowledge a philosopher needs for comprehensive understanding of the world and self" (Bergson in Murphy 1994).

Intuition means "to receive knowledge by direct perception. ... the mind's immediate apprehension of an object without the intervention of any reasoning process." Insights

Chapter 8

lie beneath and beyond the rational mind – they are *felt* coming from within. When lucid we catch them unfolding. Wisdom is there, waiting patiently for acknowledgment.

Insight may arise from instinct and intuition founded on:

- a protoself

- archaic consciousness

- mythical or magical consciousness

- subliminal consciousness

- the acknowledgment of spatial consciousness

- the activity of dynamic consciousness

- the fact that we can see a deeper reality as the ego yields.

Creative emptiness

Knowing without content arises as we pass through sensations of creative engagement and follows *knowing with content* which is in itself an insight. Personal insight is fertilized within inner space. Spiritual teachers might propose that insight has been there from the beginning as an aspect of universal consciousness and wisdom. Our spiritual reason for being may be to download and channel insight. Physical sensation and spatial consciousness unite materiality with nonmateriality to produce a profound source of insight and realization.

Physicist David Bohm comments:

it is held that the more complex an animal the greater its display of intelligence, but the intelligence must also be immanent in the matter that constitutes the animal. If the immanence is pursued more and more deeply in matter, I believe we may

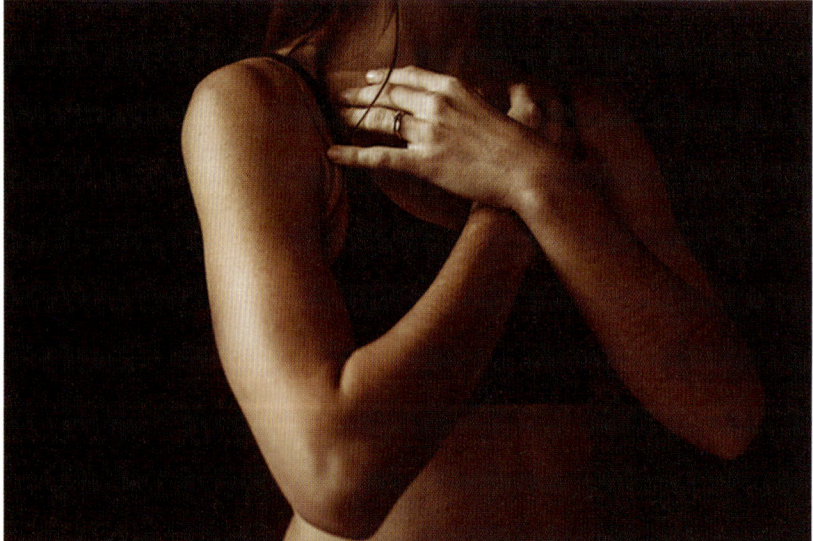

Personal insight arises from the fertility of inner space. Spiritual teachers might say that insight has been there from the beginning as an aspect of universal consciousness and wisdom. Our spiritual reason for being may be to download and channel the energy of universal insight.

INSIGHT AND WISDOM

eventually reach the stream which we also experience as mind, so that mind and matter fuse. We call the ultimate heights of mind transcendence; we find in the depths of matter the immanence of the whole of that which is. (Bohm in Wilber 1982)

Bohm's statement may point to the ultimate source of insight. Deep sensory experience transcends into insightful consciousness.

The more profound the realization, the more irrepressible the need to share it. Insight materializes into thought words, and we deliver these in a language that gives them form. "The eternal forms cannot be perceived with the senses, but grasped only by intellectual intuition. This intuition is not reached by mere thinking, but by mystical insight" (Sheldrake 2011). Rupert Sheldrake may be correct, but we sense it in our bodies, before and as the intellectual intuition assimilates the meaning. The body opens for the intellectual expression of insight.

We can be filled with ideas on how to do and what to feel, an ongoing analysis of how we experience our work. This is expected as part of the learning process but dampens the spatial lucidity that produces insight and realization. Creative emptiness arrives when we are free from the constraints of *how and what*. The *idea* of emptiness is a step in the right direction and yields to emptiness itself. Emptiness creates the clarity for emergent insight.

Letting it out

Sharing insight requires trust in our experience. Am I qualified to articulate such deep realizations? Who am I to say these things? "Who am I?" may be more to the point, as an unfamiliar part of oneself comes to the surface. At some point personal insight should be trusted. Secondhand observations are safe but limiting. Growth as a teacher involves exposing our authenticity. Letting it out is a part of the process. Confidence in sharing our insights teaches us more about teaching than anything else.

Insight has no place on a class plan. Should we have an insight beforehand, it may go down well with the group but lacks the energy of an on-the-spot realization while "we are in it together." In one way it has all been said before. Everyone is saying the same thing: one truth, one vastness, and so on. But we may not have *felt* it, expressed its embodiment, and shared it in our own words. Each time we do, we grow in some way. *Insightfulness* as an ongoing state is an indication that we have transcended the impediments of rational consciousness.

Personal insight can be supported by what others have said. We might refer to traditional yoga, Eastern thought, psychology, psychoanalysis, or quantum physics. If we have studied along these lines, these aspects will be revealed in some way anyway. This aside, we can let out personal observations, free from the philosophy, science, or spiritual insight of others. We ride our own observations, are responsible for our words, and must trust the consequences. Spiritual teachers have said many things based on extraordinary insight. We hear these gratefully but gain little by adding them to a current enlightening experience. We feel the experience in our bodies, and it springs from our own consciousness and intuition. Spontaneous realizations are uncontainable They can take us by surprise and, when they do, can inspire others.

Chapter 8

> As you feel an insight build catch it softly. The words find themselves and escape into the room. There is no spiritual guide to support you, only you, seeing the insight, letting it out. Feel your energy change. Confidence follows clarity. The group merges into a field of realization.

The inner sage

Insightful experience dissolves the ego. We have this experience on a regular basis. We could be modern mystics investing in the unknown and engaging with possibilities that are free from completion. Mystical experience gains insight into the nature of existence without conclusion. Sages over the centuries have come to the conclusion of inconclusiveness. They have also pointed out that we should find this realization in and for ourselves. A conclusion reached by addressing our conditioned ego. We have an inner sage! Sagacity is a state, a bottom line from which wisdom *about* something can materialize. Wisdom is a gentle flowing movement founded on instinct and intuition. *Wisdom is defined as the capacity of judging rightly in matters relating to life and conduct and sound sense* and as *knowledge of a high or abstruse kind*. Abstruse refers to the mysterious. The term *philosophy* is derived from two Ancient Greek words: *philo*, meaning love, and *sophia*, meaning wisdom. If we love wisdom, we are philosophers. Wisdom defines qualities such as insight, understanding, farsightedness, knowing, perception, intelligence, and common sense.

Other people's wisdom can be inspiring, but it is not our wisdom. Over-reliance on the wisdom of others and continually quoting their words is philosophical and spiritual laziness. Emergent wisdom formulates from *our* perceptions into *our* words and, although resonant with the wisdom of others, remains authentically *ours*. We *feel* wisdom first hand. Others may set a *bar* of wiseness and draw attention to the possibilities, but beyond a point the wisdom of others stops us moving and inhibits authentic sagacity.

Wisdom is associated with such attributes as unbiased judgement, compassion, experiential self-knowledge, self-transcendence and nonattachment. Wisdom is an intelligence that is also described as a penetration, presumably the penetration of the fog of habit and conditioning in order to reveal clarity and some inner truth.

Where does wisdom come from and how does it arise? Wisdom is suffocated by conditioning. The body has a wisdom that is reflected by its intelligence. Working with sensation enhances wisdom generally by helping to dissolve conditioned patterns of behavior.

There is a wisdom about nothing in particular, the wisdom of insight and realization, and a wisdom for the sake of itself. In group work we can highlight the wisdom of space and silence that leads us toward authentic and profound teaching.

A common wisdom

The essential wisdom of life is common sense. We might find as much common sense in our neighborhood as anywhere in the East. The depth of homegrown common sense might

Insight and Wisdom

be so familiar it defies acknowledgment or celebration. We see things as they are and act accordingly. Like most things of deeper value, it is unclear where common sense comes from. It may be a positive side of conditioning or spring from the ego's integration with subliminal consciousness. Common sense feels like a fundamental awareness merging with the ability to discern and evaluate. A chemistry of common sense might show an absence of adrenaline and sympathetic activity and a predominance of oxytocin and parasympathetic activity. Wisdom is not flushed with excitement or tinged with stress or anxiety but is rich in calmness and kindness.

Common sense, "the people's wisdom" (folk wisdom), is defined as an *unreflective knowledge not reliant on specific training or deliberative thought.* Common sense is distinct from basic sensory perception and rational thinking but cooperates with both. Some people have well-established common sense before they start yoga and may risk losing it by immersing in an extreme philosophy or practice beyond common sense. We can flavor common sense with an Eastern philosophy and inject common sense into an Eastern philosophy. We can view sensory awareness as a physiological common sense that influences the wisdom of common sense. Immersion into a *common sensory field* unveils the common sensibilities underlying the quality of the process. It is a sense in the true sense of the word!

Common sense implies good sense in practical issues and communication. We need common sense to hold and guide groups. This includes an acknowledgment that each person has their own guiding principle, a degree of common sense. Suggestions, insights, and possibilities need a common-sense delivery. Common sense addresses the realities of life and constructs words to describe mystical possibilities. Mysticism is one of life's realities.

Wisdom:

- thrives on a stable, calm sense of self

- is enhanced by dissolving conditioning and deepening perception

- emanates from the body as a sensation

- feels like a gentle, outward flowing movement

- emerges with a heightening sensitivity and awareness

- is dynamized by the appropriate physical sensations

- reflects an ancient relationship between the energy of living tissue and the energy of knowing

- is an intelligence that surfaces in the presence of physical, psychological, and emotional space

- reflects a human tendency to give to ourselves and to others.

Wisdom can be found anywhere and in anyone. Children are inherently wise (out of the mouths of babes), their wisdom

Chapter 8

uncontaminated by the conditioning of life experience. You may recall being put to bed early as a child, not being sleepy, gazing out of the window when it was still light outside, and innocently *knowing* the nature of existence. (Theta brain waves, predominant in meditation, are also predominant in young children.)

Together, as a group, we return to where we once were, a state of flowing innocence and wonder, engaging with a field of wisdom. Emergent wisdom is an intelligence, it holds and unites us, and has more to do with a way of being than a given situation, although the former informs the latter. We are personally and collectively wise.

The wisdom of choice

As teachers, we are faced with the choices around how best to frame current experience as it arises. The word *intelligence* means *to choose between* and is derived from the Latin words *inter,* meaning *between,* and *ligo,* meaning *choose.* Choosing is an essential intelligence. Choosing is wisdom in action. When we are in the thick of it with a group we cannot predict a choice in advance. Common sense chooses descriptions that favor the most positive outcomes. We can choose whether to focus on sensation or consciousness. We choose when to speak, when to remain silent, when to listen to our self, and when and how to bring the group toward our experience. We can choose to slow things down and give time to sense anxiety, flux, or distraction in the group. We can choose to take the practice in another direction. We should be clear on choices. It is not uncommon to bounce between intelligent and less intelligent choices.

At any given time we may choose between the words space, softness, or lightness to hold the attention of the group. The choice comes from the nature of the session at the time, and could involve aspects related to tissue tension, states of mind, expansion, or anything within the spectrum of current experience. Choosing to slow down more than we think we need to magnifies awareness and gives an opportunity to make more intelligent choices generally.

Choosing intelligently is the beginning of *choicelessness.* It is a way of being that is not influenced by shifts in tissue tension or mental activity. We can also choose between choosing and choicelessness and allow everything to pass through the proverbial stream of consciousness. Choicelessness is the companion of emptiness. All things unfold as they will.

Another confidence

An insight is a condensation of wisdom. Authentic insight produces an innovative narrative because there is no previous language to describe it. We can easily quote the Buddha or relate an experience to a sutra, but quotations inhibit the immediate effect of an insight.

Allowing an insight to fly requires the confidence to let it out. Then it is gone, it is out there. Sustaining a flow of wisdom requires faith in our ongoing perceptions and presence of mind. Trusting personal wisdom requires another kind of confidence. Wisdom at best implies insightfulness, a continuum of realization, and a state or condition with the fertility for a specific

INSIGHT AND WISDOM

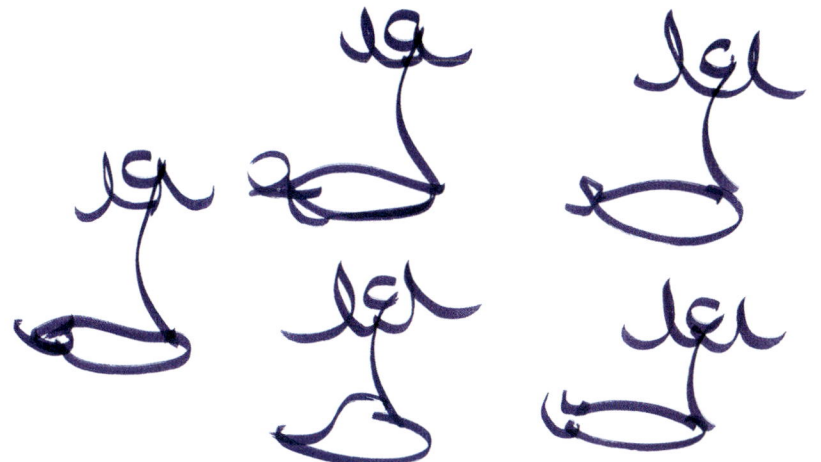

> As we bring the group back, as they process, we can elaborate on an insight or highlight the nature of understanding without content.

insight should it materialize. Insightfulness is akin to the condition of *knowing*, free from pervasive thought, and is a wisdom that holds a group, inspires their confidence, and gives freedom for discovery. Confidence comes as we channel wisdom and trust that students take what they need.

The feeling of understanding

Insight and wisdom stem from an *underlying* feeling of *understanding*. Consciousness houses a *feeling* of understanding. The basic *feeling* of understanding is a state needing neither content nor subject. Wisdom begins with a sense of understanding nothing in particular.

Understanding is taken from the Old English *understandan*, taken literally meaning *stand in the midst of*, and is related to Middle High German, meaning *to stand in front of, under, or beneath*. Understanding is the essence of intelligence. *Understanding* as a sense moves with consciousness and suggests a *knowing* that provides the basis for insight and wisdom. As with consciousness and knowing, understanding is embodied. Expansive sensations draw us into the feeling of understanding. In the same way that we *come* to an understanding *with* someone or *about* something we can be brought back *to* the quality of understanding without content.

Insight and wisdom are grounded in a reflective feeling of understanding in conjunction with the general experience of life. The energy supporting insight and wisdom arises from a primal consciousness that is formulated and expressed as a sense, with or without content, depending upon the needs of the moment. A sense of understanding is an intelligence that feeds all intelligence and supports common sense. A *field* of understanding pervades a practicing group and sets the scene for authentic insight. The sagacity of sages, the seeing of seers, and the wisdom of wise ones are implicit. We can share insight with others while inviting them to acknowledge their own realizations.

Chapter 8

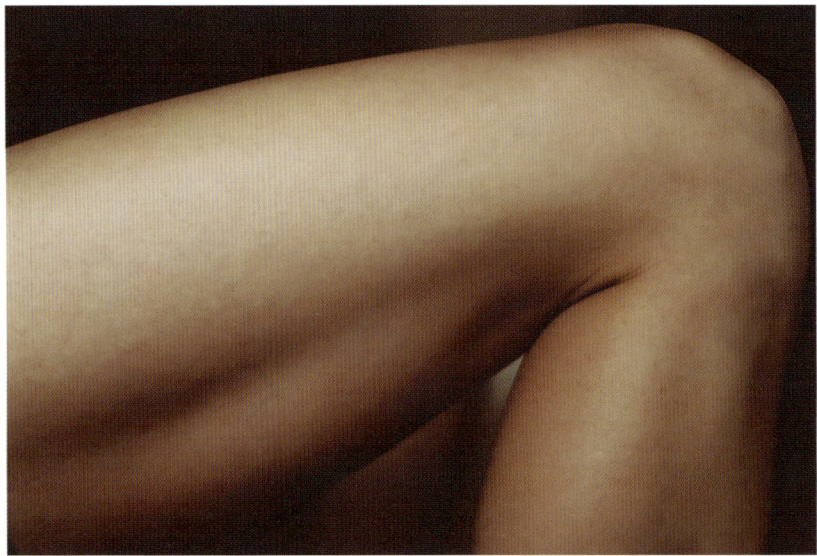

Emerging insights happen and leave spontaneously. Their expression frees us, but we may be left with an additional trace of wisdom.

Enter an area of tissue and wait for expansion. As expansion spreads, take note of what comes to mind. Sense a feeling of wisdom in your body. If and when an insight emerges, accept it. If alone, write it down. If with a group, share it. See where it leads.

Stalling

An unfolding wisdom does not guarantee immunity from misjudgment. We might see it coming. Internal slips may or may not be externalized. The timing or pace of a creative expression may be misjudged. We can all stall and attempt to fill the space. The awakened sensitivity of the group may highlight the discordance. Slowing down and riding the gentle wave of understanding reduces the impulse to act. We may be processing our experience as the group processes theirs. Teaching can be at its best when we rise to the challenge of the unexpected and channel it into productive expression. Declaring that we have stalled can bond a group even more, but this requires another confidence at a time when confidence may be scarce.

Let the experience be enough. Be content with light engagement and soft sensation. It takes very little to initiate a flow of energy throughout the surface of the body, one that touches the deepest areas and spreads out into the surrounding space. Wait and see what comes to mind. Share the outcome using your lightest and calmest voice.

Settling and receiving

Settling into a deeper understanding passes through sensation, ongoing activity, and spiritual ideas. Every "thing" is a stage from

Insight and wisdom

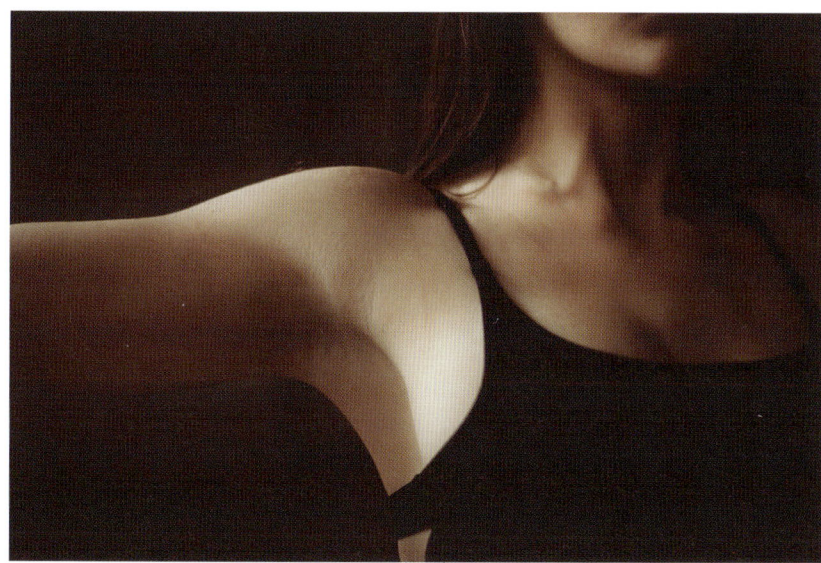

> Insight is more dynamic than the physical practice that releases it. Insight is dynamized by the reach of its field.

which the next leap of consciousness projects us toward creative emptiness. Receiving an undisturbed flow of awareness invites insightfulness. The ultimate wisdom is found in receptive space. Court the space around your perceptions, actions, and choices. Insight is more dynamic than the physical practice that releases it. Insight is dynamized by the reach of its field.

Esoteric philosophy and practice is an attempt to understand ourselves in relation to the bigger picture. In the process we are given access to insights and realization. We may return to a time before conditioning took hold. I am the same person I was at 10, 20, and 30 years old. I have the same core perceptions and understanding. Insight has been there from the beginning. It is no coincidence that wisdom flows with love, that love is the essential wisdom, and is in itself an insight. Our continuance is based on the wisdom of bonding and love. Expansion releases oxytocin and love. Oxytocin is the hormone of wisdom.

Insights are not always spiritual realizations but may be common-sense observations regarding the nature of existence and our part in it. Insights may touch on what yoga is, what the yoga masters meant, or they may consider the Western approach to conditioning, our limitations, and our potential. As we bring the group back (out of a posture, a way of being) as they process, we might elaborate on a current insight, share an understanding, and invite feedback.

The art

We cannot construct insights, impose wisdom, or learn to be insightful or wise (although being around wisdom is productive). Wisdom comes from direct experience. Life experience instills practical wisdom but the condition of wisdom is *understood* through inner experience. Quoting others may support our experience but the reality is ours. Emerging insights

Chapter 8

happen and then leave. We are set free by their expression and left with an additional trace of wisdom.

There is an art to remaining free while the mind formulates a self-made parable that makes you want to reach for your pen. We can value our words without attachment and let go of emergent insight by sharing it. Moments of deep wisdom are usually based on the same unitive theme. Opening the skin over the heart feels like cosmic grace.

Creative sensation stimulates a creative mind, awakens consciousness, and releases insight. The combination of heightened sensation and undisturbed composure brings a lucid sensitivity. Sensations are enlightening, but *lucid emptiness* transcends sensation. The sensation of space – the feeling of *hardly being there* – indicates we are transcending our body and approaching pure consciousness. The sense of space and uncluttered penetrative consciousness enter into each other.

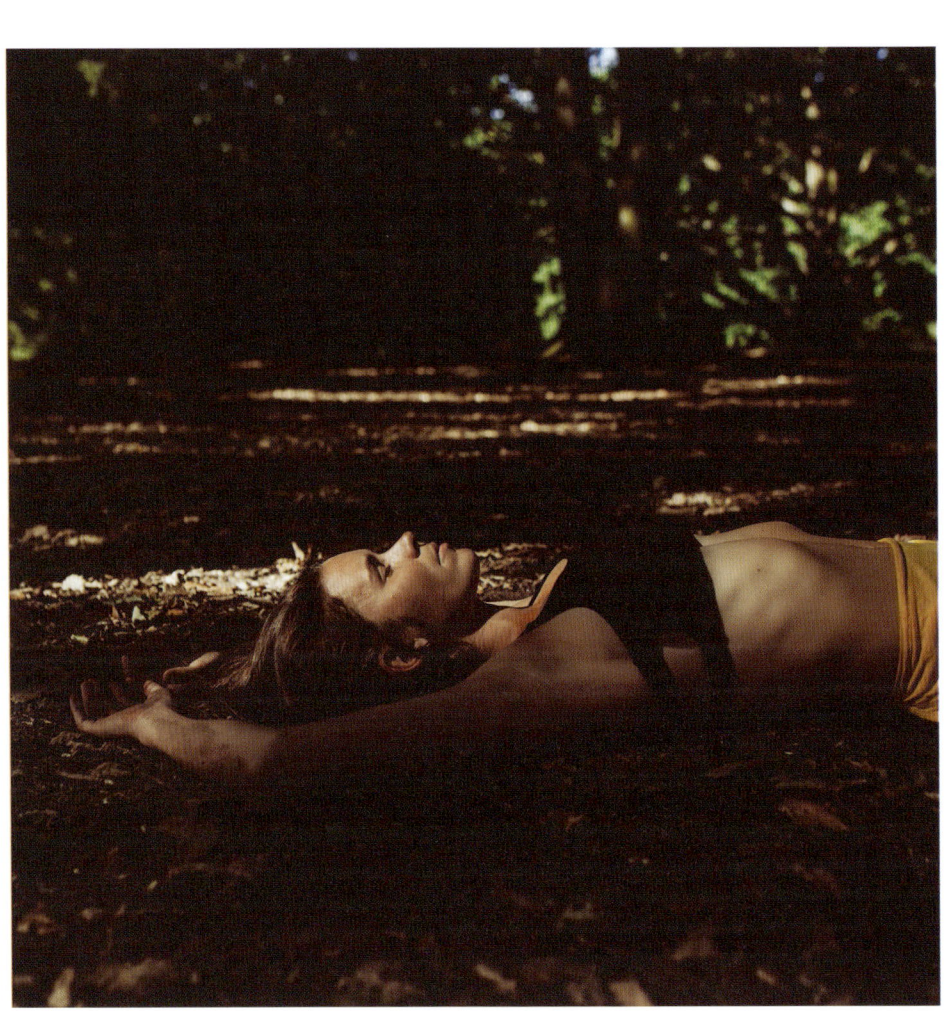

Authentic teaching

Teaching from immediate experience requires an authentic creativity, an indelible sense of the present, and an intuitive ability for detecting moment-to-moment needs. We arrive at a shared place through personal creativity. Individuality promotes authenticity. Authenticity is the degree to which our actions are consistent with our experience and understanding.

The word *authentic* implies *acting on one's own authority*. The word *author* comes from the Latin *auctor* meaning literally *one who causes to grow*. Teachers usually start with a given method and develop it to suit personal creativity or move beyond it entirely. Listening more closely to our body–mind compels us to teach from our own discoveries while refining or transforming an accepted structure. There are only so many ways a body can be positioned or move, and beyond that there are extensive, ever-changing permutations we can refer to. Given one mind, its kaleidoscopic activity can be forged into clear and present insight. We can *cause others to grow* from the inspiration that comes from our own growth. There is a broad spectrum between what someone has shown us and listening to the ever-changing richness of a sensory system expressing its creative intelligence. The field is wide open for refining sensation, consciousness, and insight. Authenticity may be based upon an initial framework from which *things happen*, but frameworks stand still. Authenticity is understanding in the making: it moves.

Authenticity arises from following spontaneous responses as we receive, convey, and let go of sensations and insights. "To some extent, *every* individual organism and every element of its structure and behaviour represents a creative response to its internal and external condition" (Sheldrake 2011).

Creativity is an upward movement from within. Jean Gebser observed:

the German word for "creative" is schöpferisch, from schöpfen, to "draw up (water)", for the creative person "draws up" from the well-springs of life … what has not yet been realized. … creativity is something that "happens" to us, that fully effects or fulfills itself in us … Through creativity preconscious origin becomes the conscious present … Since creativity is a potency or

Chapter 9

energy it cannot be grasped systematically ... it is a potency which only rarely manifests in its full strength. (Gebser 1949/1985)

Gebser was aware that enabling deeper consciousness was a creative act. Awakened creativity becomes known to consciousness but the process occurs beneath awareness. We can see the consequences of creativity but cannot see a material representation of the nature of creativity. Creativity occurs. Our practices prepare us for a creativity that happens to us. For us, creativity is an unbound entity that dances between sensation, mental activity, and consciousness. Gebser's suggestion that potency rarely manifests in its full strength may apply to those whose creativity needs time to accept the impact of dynamic consciousness. Others may engage with the power of dynamic consciousness while being creatively expressive. Sharing an alternative consciousness with a group is a creative act.

The great yoga scholar Georg Feuerstein wrote:

Human creativity then unfolds at the interface between consciousness and the hidden dimension of the mind ... It draws on higher-order faculties while at the same time yielding to the promptings of the submerged part of the psyche: the unconscious or subconscious. Whatever universal features it may have, it always represents a unique personal gesture, calling for an unstinting investment of the creative individual's energies and thus a singular kind of courage. (Feuerstein 1997)

It can take courage to broadcast a surge of insight. As creativity surfaces, each word is considered and chosen creatively. Censorship and choice determine the quality of the words that express emerging realizations.

Creative awareness

We create a field of change by awakening sensory and mental experience. Creative intelligence arises from a mysterious source and is stimulated by our attention. Sheldrake writes: "But why should matter, energy, life or process be creative? This is inevitably mysterious. Not much more can be said than it is their nature to be so" (Sheldrake 2011). *Why* we are creative may or may not be of interest, but *how* to be creative is the key to authentic teaching. We are recreating ourselves and inviting others to do likewise within a cocreative field of possibility. There are various avenues through which creativity can express itself. Here are just some that we can tap into and use during practice and teaching.

Sensory creativity

The creative impulse occurs in the space between sensation and realization. Once expressed, we return to the wellspring of the spatial unknown. Sustaining sensory attention creates an awareness that replenishes itself with insight. We express sensation with a measured commentary. Tissue activity creates and recreates deeper levels of understanding. Countless sensory nerve endings receive and transmit information between the surface and depths of the body. We can consciously dance with sensation. Sensory creativity comes from listening to and following sensation. This level of interaction fine-tunes the mind and gives access to the

AUTHENTIC TEACHING

deeper reaches of consciousness. Advanced sensations appeal to the finer aspects of sensory activity. Insights and realizations are also sensations but are inhibited by the background activity we may be unaware of.

> Sense a change of texture between your skin and the underlying fascia and between soft tissue and bone. Sense the continuity of the skin as one entire piece. Allow the sensations to pass through awareness. Follow the movement of tissue as it opens from one area to the next. Create a commentary that describes the experience.

Mechanical creativity

The creative space between mechanical sensation and consciousness is open to suggestion. Suggesting width or length brings width or length. How does this happen? It is a question that physiology cannot answer, at least not the final step between the suggestion and the experience. An unknown intelligence is at work. Sensing required mechanical relationships inspires us to position and organize the spine, limbs, and girdles to promote involuntary responses. Creativity explores the finer movements of the limbs in relation to the shoulder and pelvic girdle and draws attention to the spinal curves. The art of mechanical creativity is in following the skeletal activity that encourages and is encouraged by the activity on the surface. Gently raising the shoulder girdle in advance of raising the arm is a creative act that softens and opens the entire upper body. Resettling the shoulder girdle before bringing the arm down is a creative act that releases all superfluous tension.

Organic creativity

Tissue responsivity reveals the organic intelligence underpinning mechanical organization. Our influence on the skeletal framework is based on our ability to read tissue sensations. We can perceive the entire body as an organic intelligence that informs and directs creativity.

The tissue of the wrists informs the tissue of the ribs, pelvis, and breastbone. Ankle tissue is felt influencing shoulder blade and neck tissue. Raising an arm can be felt over the surface of the thighs. The movements of the breath include tissue responses throughout the whole body. Simply being attentive to an area of tissue provokes a subtle and expansive response. Tissues move and respond in countless ways. The surface of the body can feel as if it slides around, part to part, and, given the freedom, moves in unpredictable ways.

The organism is self-stimulating and, when awakened, awakens the mind to an awakened consciousness.

Respiratory creativity

Creative intelligence serves the moment-to-moment chemical needs of the tissues. The

Chapter 9

breath is naturally creative when undisturbed by our intervention. Breathing supports and is supported by mechanical and organic intelligence. Waiting at the end of an exhale invites respiratory intelligence to attract an inhalation at the precise moment it is needed, something we cannot know in advance. The slightest anticipation disturbs the breath's natural creativity. We can stand back to the extent that it hardly feels like the breath, just a sliver of understated sensory activity passing through spatial consciousness. The respiratory diaphragm can feel like a creature having an independent agenda. It knows how to reset itself and may behave in ways that appear to have no bearing on the gross activity of inhaling and exhaling. If a more expansive breath is needed, the body will take it.

Fluid creativity

The distribution of fluids is a creative process sensed as a softening liquidity throughout the body. The subtle hydrodynamics of cerebrospinal fluid distribution, although not fully understood, have invaluable effects on how we feel. Fluid can be drawn into expansion, along with tissue and consciousness, as a part of the overall feeling of being drawn into space. Fluid molecules have space between them. Space is the connective tissue of fluid. When our attention is drawn to fluid sensation, it changes, deepens, and expands its spread.

Emotional creativity

The registration of emotions such as love, compassion, disappointment, excitement, and joy comes from an intelligence that drives behavior and *creates* action. We cannot organize our emotions or switch them on or off, but we can improve our relationship to them by surrounding them with space. Noticing how we feel is a creative process. Acknowledging the feeling dissolves the emotions *about* the emotion. Do you notice your emotions as you teach? A significant range of feelings can go unnoticed because of the focus on the group.

When you are aware of the emotions that lie behind the mask of the teacher and when you put space around them, the quality of the field changes. Language becomes more considered and depth more profound. Emotional creativity is found in the calm space we give to our feelings. Insight and wisdom surface as primary emotions.

Spiritual creativity

If we know how spirituality feels, and what it is, we might engage with it creatively. It is useful to look at what others have said if only to discover how spiritual we are. Spirituality arises as conditioning fades (unless we are spiritually conditioned). We have a spiritual core dating back to, and probably prior to, magical and mythical consciousness. Groups draw out spiritual experiences as if we are returning to a time before ego development, a time of wonder and amazement. In its purest form spirituality is an energized emptiness, a fullness free from content. Spatial and dynamic consciousnesses are spiritually creative!

AUTHENTIC TEACHING

Jean Gebser cites an ancient Chinese statement:

Creativity is the "primal power" which is light-giving, active, strong, and of the spirit ... Its energy is represented as unrestricted by any fixed conditions in space and is therefore conceived of as motion. ... Creativity in man is an effectualization of the creative in the world. The creativity of the world or the "heaven" is genuine or primary, whereas that of man is secondary. (Gebser 1949/1985)

Expansion is a spiritual experience. In the absence of an external stimulus we can discover an inner source of spirituality. Inherent spirituality residing in consciousness is made conscious.

Dissolving conditioned behavior deepens spiritual experience. At its simplest, spirituality is unification.

We can create a field and a form of expression that invites others toward a spiritual experience.

Ego creativity

The ego, although prone to conditioning and indiscretion, can orchestrate creativity. The ego (the I am) continually creates and recreates itself from deep roots, steering expediency, overseeing behavior, identifying emotional and spiritual experience, and, where necessary, discarding intellectualization. The ego transforms itself by recognizing and guiding the creative impulse. The most productive teaching is guided by an ego that listens to itself and to everything entering its experience. The ego responds to an ancient egolessness as it registers sensory changes in density and continuity. The ego registers the nature of consciousness and directs itself accordingly. It acknowledges shifts in behavior, as sensation informs

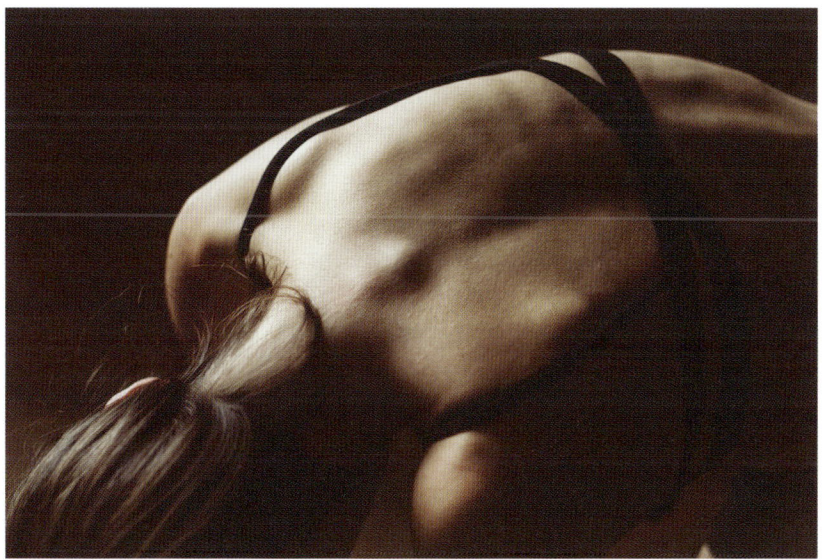

In its purest form spirituality manifests as an energized emptiness, a fullness free from content.

Chapter 9

consciousness and consciousness informs itself. The ego in pure unconditioned form is inseparable from consciousness and at the same time is the actor. A group is made up of separate egos acknowledging personal experiences that flow into and receive from the group ego. The "I am" and the "we are" meet cocreatively.

Intellectual creativity

An aspect of intelligence, the intellect, is subservient to the ego and responsible for creative thought, ideas, and constructs. The intellect has the capacity for knowledge and objective understanding in relation to abstract matters. We use the intellect to discuss the yoga experience and underpin debate. Training courses could not function in the absence of creative intellectualization. We knowingly intellectualize experiences that may be beyond intellectualization. We use the intellect to describe and analyze sensory activity and the depth of consciousness. We intellectually acknowledge tissue activity, variable selves, and the scope of teaching while sharing an unbounded experience.

Creative consciousness

Consciousness as such is not creative in terms of the usual meaning of the word creative. Consciousness is *in creation. It recreates itself from moment to moment. It unfolds.*

Our creativity is an expression *around* the constancy and clarity of dynamic consciousness, which although stemming from organic activity is found within it.

In this respect pure and lucid consciousness provides the potential for profound creativity. Observing the mind's tendency to change direction, its unpredictability, and its potential for reintegration is a creative act springing from an undeterred consciousness. Everything that is available to consciousness is subject to the creative instinct. As consciousness extends in depth more possibilities arise. We can follow consciousness as it opens, expands, and penetrates all aspects of its own content. "Creativity to the extent that it takes place in man is effected in the formation of consciousness" (Gebser 1949/1985). We can be creative with consciousness itself. To do so involves taking charge of and engaging with consciousness. We can apply the mind to consciousness in the same way that we apply the mind to tissue sensation. We can learn how to feel the quality of consciousness. We can invite others to do likewise. Together we can explore the fact of consciousness.

Creativity and conditioning

Creativity emerges as conditioning lifts. In turn, creativity addresses conditioning as we awaken to our internal behavior. A *self* is a creative process subject to the unpredictability of conditioning. We can be conditioned and creative. Conditioning can produce all kinds of creativity. Whereas artists may create to break through the restraints of their conditioning, our spatially creative consciousness can observe the nature of conditioning within itself. Inner creativity observes the nature of conditioning.

Authentic Teaching

We awaken to an inner creativity through the behavioral shifts and insights that change and inform our teaching.

Authentic choice

Choice is a creative act. Behavior is transformed by *creatively noticing*. The first choice is choosing to notice. We can become increasingly sensitive to the finer balance between too much or too little tension and we can highlight the delicate nature of texture and subtle ways of being. Creativity makes choices but not all choices are intelligent. Well-trodden paths do not dissolve readily. We can choose expansion and silence or not. Students understand the simplicity of choice and learn to turn away from unwanted reactions.

Yoga advocates the nonduality of choiceless awareness. It takes time to get to this point and takes longer to learn how to sustain it. Along the way we find ourselves between opposing ways of being. We can choose between a contractive reaction or a gentle and expansive response. Students can be drawn into conditioned responses throughout an entire practice without realizing that they are doing so. Feeling refreshed after a class is beneficial but does not shift the deeper patterns. We can impose a practice onto a lifetime's investment in conditioned behavior or we can choose not to. We can learn and teach how to choose our experience.

We choose wisely when we slow right down and keep the space open. Choosing expansion draws the mind out of itself. Individual interpretations of the same experience can differ but a shift in consciousness pervades the group. As density dissolves, the material and nonmaterial aspects of experience coalesce. Sensation, emotion, spirituality, and consciousness unite.

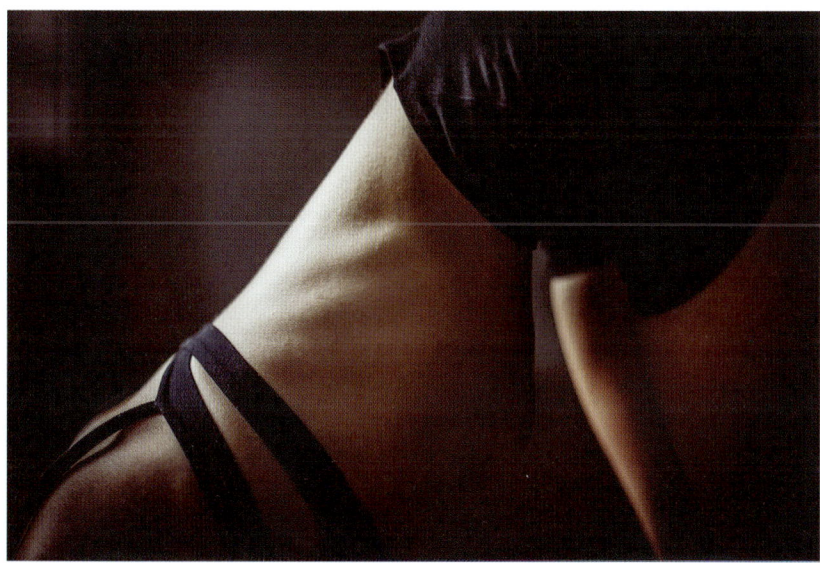

Each moment might present a choice. We choose wisely when we slow right down and keep the space open.

Chapter 9

Describing experience

Nothing is as powerful as the spoken word.
—Rudyard Kipling

Language has made a contribution to the evolution of the mind. We are creative with words, the space between them, and their direction of focus. We creatively describe and depict our own experience and suggest the same possibilities to others. The word *depict* means *to portray in words, to give a graphic account of*. *Graphic* means *vividly descriptive and lifelike*. We teach through the "vivid and lifelike" use of words.

Words combined with heightened sensation have a profound effect. Words hold a group's attention, can sustain an egoless state, and can facilitate a transformative experience. Words enhance personal experience and the group field.

Nouns are weak transmitters. Words such as floor, wall, foot, or pelvis are dead on their own. They have no movement. Nouns are necessary to give direction but lack the impact of adjectives such as light, soft, deep, and spacious. Adjectives that describe nouns are effective, for example, light shoulders, soft pelvis, and so on. Verbs in the present tense have the most impact because they are actively fluid in the now. *Spreading, deepening, opening, expanding*, and *knowing* are good examples.

Space between words or sentences gives time for the ego to assimilate the suggestions and convert them into direct experience. Spatial consciousness places words into perspective and moulds them to suit current experience.

Bringing everyone into a cohesive field is a creative act. Authenticity may spring from our preconscious or from deeper roots: *where did that come from?* As the creative impulse surfaces, there may be a loss of self between the feeling of understanding and the words used to express it. And then they have it: the words dissolve into the group experience, to return again as a heightened sense or an insight.

> In the group's deepest moments share the acknowledgment of a creative presence. Surrender to a language that describes the experience.

Projection and presence

Projecting our experience is an art. A *projection* is defined as a *mental image visualized and regarded as an objective reality*. The word *projective* is defined as *the quality of being mentally projected or the power of projecting*. We are projectors, consciously projecting sensation and understanding onto and into a group's experience. We project sensation, insight, and lucid consciousness. Projection is a deliberate working tool arising from a strong sense of self. Self-presence is the center of a teacher's field. Experiencing our personal presence as a material element is the starting point. The depth of a teacher's presence ignites group receptivity. Actors, performers, speakers, and teachers project their presence. Presence is a silent language that combines containment and expansion. A core of containment radiates into the surrounding space. We unfold for the benefit of the group.

AUTHENTIC TEACHING

Presences differ

- *Unrefined presence* has little self-awareness, sensitivity, or self-reflection. *Unrefined presence* is ungenerous, cannot project, and can have a nonunitive and inhibitive effect on others.

- *Reflective presence* has a contained self-awareness and a sense of *knowing*. It is aware of the group but mainly in terms of itself. *Reflective presence* projects by default. The group is an extension of the teacher's ego and receives guidance in a limited way through their own receptivity. Reflective presence impedes the transmission of fields.

- *Harmonious presence* is refined, generous, all-encompassing, co-operative, self-reflective, and group-reflective. *Harmonious presence* introduces and sustains a sensitivity to the totality of the occasion. It projects as a continual movement, and gives the space and support for others to make discoveries for themselves. Transformative shifts occur during harmonious presence.

> Go inward and sense the relationship between your inner space and the receptivity of the group. Consciously project your sense of self as an extension of your inner space, physical sensation, and conscious awareness. Begin guidance from an outflowing all-encompassing presence.

Originality

The inseparability of living tissue and consciousness invites an original meditation. The meditation is inherent: it springs from the realization of *what is*. The term "what is" implies the blend of two sensitivities: a sensitivity to a complete sense of self and a sensitivity to the totality of life. "What is" cannot be *applied* as a meditation because "what is" lies beneath the veneer of conditioned reality. We have "what is" with or without yoga and had it as children. Some may have called it daydreaming, and perhaps it was. Perhaps it was the soul attempting to reset itself in response to what was going on around and within us.

We can summon the source of lucid consciousness by going into tissue presence and texture. Tissue cannot be pinned down and is free to open, move, shift, and behave as it will. Following tissue behavior creates an endless source of creative realization. In turn, the combination of tissue sensation and mental fluctuation is taken up and dissolved by spatial and dynamic consciousness.

On one level behavior is just activity. We can let activity pass by with little if any reference to its content. But a release *from* content enables consciousness to reorganize itself. We may be left with an ocean of consciousness. Perhaps we merge with a quantum sea of energy. Thoughts become like stars within a vast universal space: small concentrations of activity without significance. Consciousness can acknowledge its depth and its sensation. The ego rests back following the expansion of skin as its residual sensation gently holds us. The source of consciousness remains a mystery. We

Chapter 9

are modern mystics sharing creative intelligence. Authentic teaching changes from moment to moment. We grow and cause to grow by tuning in to current experience. Teacher and group grow together.

Krishnamacharya would teach a posture, followed by the meaning of a sutra (Desikachar & Krusche 2014). Many teach in this way. An alternative could be to engage with the sensations and then express one's own authentic insight. Authenticity implies being true to oneself. Authenticity, as mentioned, is the degree to which our actions are consistent with our experience and understanding. Authenticity is originality and our personal truth. Our truly creative moments arise when we sustain the space for authenticity to proliferate. Creative space *sees* clearly from a distance and acts from there. Spatial authenticity takes in sensation, thought, insight, consciousness, oneself, and others simultaneously.

When we invite a group to suspend their certainty by suspending our own certainty, an authentic and creative relationship can flourish.

Authentic teaching takes charge of the group and holds the space for their own experience to prevail. Space is authentic because it has no knowable content and therefore no apparent history or memory. There are various ways of doing. They may be authentically ours or borrowed. Each time we transcend them we discover and rediscover one way of being.

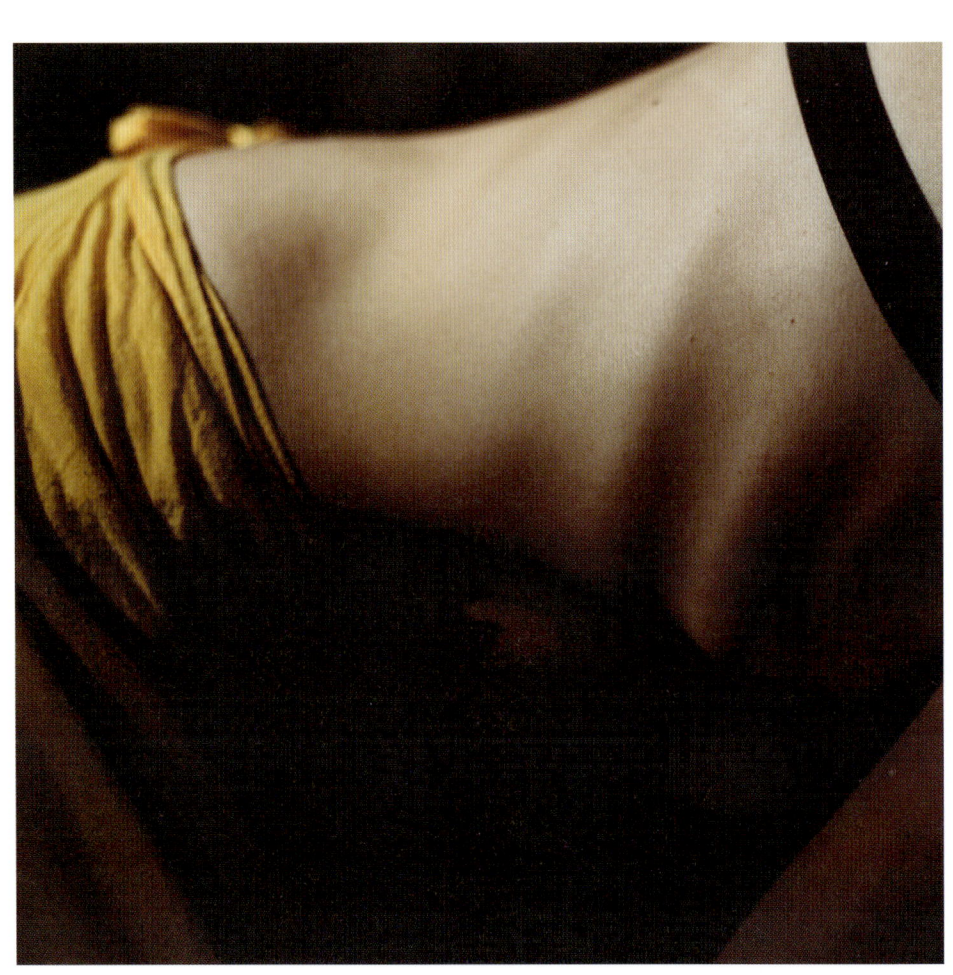

Unification

We are unifiers, providing others with the tools for realizing a profound sense of unity. The aim of yoga is not only to unify body, mind, and spirit but also to point the way to a profound and lucid unification of consciousness. We guide people through their inner space, and they move outward into a more universal experience.

Experiencing

Some things are so obvious and so continuously present that they are easily overlooked. We can take our most enriching aspect, our own embodied experience, for granted. The impulse to learn and feel may overwhelm immediate experience.

Trusting our experience, and inviting others to trust theirs, provides the bedrock for learning and teaching. Acknowledging the *fact* of experiencing is the first step. The experience of others should be acknowledged with sensitivity.

Nothing has changed since Deane Juhan wrote: "The truth of the matter is that physiologists and psychiatrists have absolutely no idea of the mechanisms which give rise to conscious experience. Nor are there any scientifically meaningful hypotheses concerning the problem" (Juhan 1987).

Whatever the factors are that conspire to provide experience, the reality that we do not know *how* experience happens enables unlimited space *for* experience. We are not tied to a physiology of experience. The neurological and biochemical route *to* experience may be understood but the jump between incoming information and the experience itself eludes scientific inquiry. An unknown space between the delivery of experience and its reception provides a key to understanding the fundamentals of yoga and meditation. The point is *that* we experience, not *how* we experience.

R. D. Laing observed:

Experience is not an objective fact. A scientific fact need not be experienced … The effect on us of an objective fact may not be an objective fact. … Total objectivity precludes itself from any possible explanation of experience. The most sophisticated neuroscientists are the most baffled at its very existence, and its inexplicable and capricious relationship to the brain. (Laing 1982)

Chapter 10

An in-depth understanding of neurophysiology has no bearing on the quality of experience. Neuroscientist Antonio Damasio writes:

I do not need to know a thing about the particular behavior of neurons and molecules in different areas of my brain in order to have the experience ... even when I recall in my mind all the knowledge of neurophysiology that I have pertinent to forming mental visual images ... it does not make one bit of difference to the forming of these current images or to my experience of them. It is nice to know a little about how the brain does its job, but it is not necessary at all to experience anything. (Damasio 2000)

For us, the experience of understanding has more relevance than understanding experience. *Experiencing* is in the present on par with *being*. Experiencing is a here-and-now involuntary movement. We can experience our own experience, experience ourselves experiencing one another, and at times can read the experience of others. Groups bond by sharing experience. Yoga suggests we should not cling to experiences. They are just experiences, within a broader field of experience: a suggestion that is difficult to adopt.

As far as we can fathom, no amount of knowledge about the neurophysiology of the formation and experience of mental images will ever produce the experience of those mental images in those who possess that knowledge, although greater knowledge will give us a more satisfactory explanation of how we come to have such experiences of images. (Damasio 2000)

Experience may be filtered through a screen of conditioning. Students may be unable to experience their conditioning but conditioning colors their experience. Yoga is *the* experiential experiment. Experience is larger than the sum of its parts. We are programmed by and for experiencing. Yoga's primary concern is how we perceive experience. Experiencing is the foundation for insight, wisdom, and understanding. A recollected experience may be useful, but *in the now experiencing* is the ever-present teacher that influences sensitivity, perception, and communication.

People understandably return to classes and workshops expecting or wanting to repeat good experiences. This expectation gives Eastern philosophy one of its basic tenets. Expecting or wanting inhibits the progressive change that happens in the present. Comparison inhibits the sense of unification. We may begin with the pleasurable memory of our last practice, but we can move on. These pleasant, or even amazing, sensory experiences, although most welcome, do not necessarily guarantee deeper shifts in consciousness. Light bulb moments may occur along the way but are no indication of more sustainable changes.

Trusting that something will come frees us for a new experience. We learn and feel more when we are not distracted by something in the past, when we are innocent. Memory impedes experiencing. Past experiences may create changes that lead to new experiences, but the movement of experience is not a finite process. Each experience is absorbed into a stream of experiencing that corresponds to an undisturbed flow of consciousness. Totality has no conclusion: it moves.

Unification

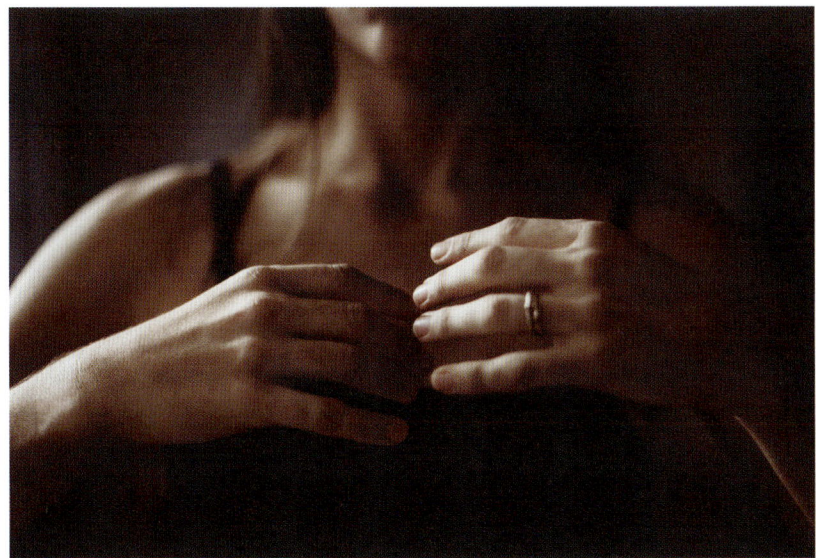

> Totality is the movement of experience, not a finite process. Each experience is unified into a movement of experiencing synonymous with an undisturbed stream of consciousness.

Deeper calm

Calmness is a quality that determines the quality of our experience. Calmness informs how we experience ourselves and one another. We should know how to switch on calmness, one of our most valuable assets. Calmness gives space to our experience and influences those within our field. Projecting ways of feeling and being requires a deepening calmness. We can be profoundly calm as a practice in itself, without the breath, meditations, or postures. Substantial, palpable calmness is rare in daily life. Considered calmness tempers the intensity of an awakening consciousness and empowers teaching. Calmness supports confidence and emotional strength. The first thing about calm is to notice that we may not be calm (enough).

Unadorned, direct calmness is a deliberate statement. We may feel calm but can slip into deeper calmness, *just like that*. It is like driving on the open road accustomed to the tone of the engine and then remembering another gear. Everything quietens down, feels smoother, and opens out.

We may deepen calm, just to see if we can. If you teach calmness and *are* calm, you may drop into more calmness. We may knowingly or unknowingly slip into a habit of less calm. "Uncalmness" is a pervasive feature of conditioning. The "uncalmness" of others can be contagious. Sustaining a deeper calm needs awareness until it becomes natural. We can sustain undisturbed calmness on meeting tension. Calmness soothes potential reactions and can radically change tissue. Beneath rational activity, within subliminal consciousness, lies a reservoir of calmness. Deep and abiding calmness is an ultimate experience that is realized once we have become *surprisingly* calmer. We can perceive calmness as an impersonal entity that arrives when we remember it.

Chapter 10

> Feel the materiality of calmness. Sense its substance. Transmit calmness. You may have one or two people in mind when referring to calmness, but a deeper calmness is taken up by everyone. Calmness holds the group. There is always another gear.

Calmness is the first and last step, an enduring and transformative element. When taken to its depth, calmness opens the door to new discoveries and heightens perception, attention, and sensitivity. We can teach and live from an enriching calmness. Some people have this naturally, but others, having practiced for years, find it elusive. Calmness is not passive but a quiet, active sense implying confidence and understanding. Calm is not only the absence of excitement or superfluous activity but also harbors lightness, knowing, and insight. Calmness is *the* adjustment, without which there is no yoga. We can start with calm. We can instill calm before anything is done or said.

We may cultivate a calm atmosphere but calmness can only be found by each person, a way of being that slips into us as we slip into it. Calmness is a presence that dissolves tension, opens sensory awareness, deepens consciousness, dissolves ambition, and brings trust and lucidity. *Essential* calmness is intensely rich, brings clarity to the entire body–mind, gives authority to our voice, and holds others in their spaciousness. Calmness dissolves the turbulence in the corners of the mind, fosters respect, and refines perception.

Calmness is an effortless, transcendent state, a background emotion moving to the foreground. Expansive action springs from calmness. The chemistry of calm takes in the chemistry of understanding, insight, and wisdom. A field of calm holds the space, the group, and the words. Calmness softens the ego and releases the quiet energy of subliminal consciousness. We can be additionally calm together, free from technique. Calmness is a natural state.

Exclusive and inclusive focus

Attention and awareness can only be authentic because we cannot use other people's attention or awareness.

Attention and *awareness* are words that we use constantly. Attention is exclusive and direct and usually focuses on a specified material or nonmaterial experience. Attention is the primary tool of consciousness and mainstay of practice. Awareness is inclusive and diffuse with a broader field. Attention and awareness overlap and feed each other. Both are perceptive and their quality relates to an awakened consciousness.

Krishnamurti's suggestion that we can transform ourselves through an immediate and attentive focus, without recourse to a practice, is a bridge too far for the majority. Immediate transformation requires unsustainable effort. It takes intense energy to penetrate established conditioning and reveal a dynamic consciousness for more than a few moments without the support of practical tools. *Attention* is defined as the *earnest direction of the mind*, while *awareness* is defined as *watchful, informed, cognizant, or conscious*. Awareness implies being aware *of* something or *having* general awareness. Awareness can

Unification

be seen as a basic space in the mind, within which all objects can be distinguished. I can be attentive *to* or aware *of* an experience.

Attention

Attention is a two-way movement. We apply our attention as a tool. We direct it and it becomes receptive. The object of our attention *comes* to our attention, it arrives. Application is the first stage and reception the next. For reception to be optimal the mind must be empty. The depth of our attention is dependent upon the receptive space in the mind.

We sustain attention at will. We can experience being attentive and are aware that attention enhances experience. Attention forges clear and vivid perception and is the bedrock of yoga. Mindfulness is attention to what is. Attention reveals spatial and dynamic consciousness.

Attention is a sense. When a creature is attentive it senses. The object of attention generates sensation. Undisturbed attention to tissue sensation magnifies and transforms the sensation. Attention involves mental vigilance applied to sensation and consciousness.

Focused attention is selective and demands total presence with its object. Distractions include other sensory stimuli, sounds, inappropriate words, ideas, emotions, and the unpredictable activity of the mind. We tend to self-distract, but can dissolve the distractions with penetrant attention and filter out what is wanted. As attention moves between sensation, consciousness, and presence, we can bring them together within a unified field. At the same time our attention divides between our experience and the experience of the group. In effect we produce a field of attention.

Attention engages with tissue and spotlights sensory aliveness and the random nuances of density and spatial activity. Attention draws us into the subtlety of all sensory and mental activity and is essential for cultivating the condition of understanding and underlying insightfulness.

Attention draws us into an ever-deepening perception and makes the distinction between what is wanted or not wanted. Attention to an experience changes the experience. Attention to *experiencing* changes its quality.

Attention has varying textures and might be hard, dull, and gripping, or light, soft, and laser like, quietly transforming its object of focus. Attention highlights the activity that invades the flow between sensation and itself. Attention observes *what happens*. At some point penetrative attention opens into an expansive awareness.

> Focus on an area of engaged tissue. Consolidate your attention to the exclusion of all else. Enter the sensation using your attention as a continual movement. Observe how the sensation yields to your attention, deepens, and then opens into a spatial sensation that blends with the space around you. The focus of attention spreads to become a dynamized awareness. We can teach while having this experience. We can harness the group's attention and draw the group into the same experience.

Chapter 10

The distractive activity that breaks into the flow between sensation and attention

↑ **Attention**

- Current life circumstances
- Highlighted irritability
- Impatience
- Sensory descriptions
- Changes of sensation
- Sensory comparisons
- Seeking previous experiences
- Foreground/background thoughts/feelings/emotions
- Other teachers
- What to teach – how to teach it
- What others have said
- Philosophical soundbites
- Eastern reference
- Anatomical/biomechanical/fascial features
- Knowledge
- Anxiety due to loss of ego
- Self-congratulation or perceived success of practice
- Holding on to personal insight

↓ **Sensation**

UNIFICATION

Awareness

Penetrative attention opens into inclusive awareness and may include everything within the field of consciousness, including consciousness itself. As attention to primary sensations opens out, we become aware of and *attend to* secondary sensations. We may start with a lateral thigh or the skin touching the floor, be drawn to the waist and then back again. Our awareness is drawn to awakening tissue and we pay attention to it. In this respect *awareness becomes attention*. Giving total attention to the skin over the pelvis releases local energy that spreads throughout the body–mind and beyond into surrounding space: *attention becomes awareness*. Consciousness is free to roam and may become larger than its content.

Attention and awareness cross over and may enhance each other. We can be aware of ourselves being attentive and be attentive to our awareness. I can be aware *of* you or attentive *to* you. I can be aware *of* someone in a group while being attentive *to* the group. Attention appears to close the mind but in effect begins to open it. Awareness may begin with a broader field but can draw down into a specific focus. Attention is a condensation of awareness, while awareness is a dispersion of that condensation. Lateral-thigh sensation belongs to a universal field.

Attention has more intensity than awareness. Attention is more effective than *intention* because conditioned patterns distort intention. If I *intend* to open tissue, the tissue is trapped by my intention. Tissue is responsive when I attend to and wait for it to change. Attention is more effective than awareness at changing tissue and penetrating habitual consciousness. Attention and awareness can only be in the present and cannot be taught but can be applied on suggestion. Our job is to sustain attention and awareness in others.

Attention and awareness coexist through a screen of conditioning. Being aware *of* and attentive *to* sensation dissolves conditioning and invites a deepening consciousness. Attention penetrates sensation and rational consciousness, while awareness identifies the need for attention. Attention and awareness are multilayered, the one becoming the other at any given moment.

I can be:

- attentive to my skin while being aware of my surroundings
- attentive to consciousness while being aware of my sensations
- attentive to primary sensations while being aware of secondary sensations
- aware of my attention and attentive to my awareness
- aware of my sensations while being attentive to the group
- aware of my words while being attentive to a field of presence
- aware of my inner space, the group, and the space between us while being attentive to the space between my words
- attentive to one person while being aware of the group
- attentive to group consciousness while being aware of my consciousness and vice versa

Chapter 10

- aware of my emotions while being attentive to the group field
- aware of the broader fabric of existence while being attentive to the group's awareness of the same.

The above is not a formula. There are endless combinations of attention and awareness driven by perception. Awareness of one's own body–mind while being attentive to the group forms the basis for *being in it with them* and produces insightful and inspired communication.

Awareness *of* tension is the first step, followed by attention *to* tension. Undisturbed penetrative attention disperses tension and opens consciousness to its own possibilities. Light and soft attention is no less penetrating and effective. Attention spreads out to become an all-encompassing intensified awareness. Attention distributes its center into expansive dynamic consciousness.

Attention, sensation, and consciousness

The senses have been a major factor in the development of consciousness and therefore of attention. Attention and consciousness have promoted the evolution of self-awareness and the knowledge that we have sensation and consciousness. Consequently, attention to sensation deepens consciousness. We go where sensation leads us. Attention to sensation deepens consciousness which in turn deepens attention. Neuroscientist Antonio Damasio suggests that stages of consciousness evolved in tandem with stages of attention. He writes: "natural low-level attention precedes consciousness, while focused attention follows the unfolding of consciousness" (Damasio 2000). He highlights the inseparability of attention and consciousness. Primitive attention underpinned ego development.

It may be a mystery exactly how and when sensation, attention, and consciousness came together. Experiencing attention's effect on sensation and consciousness is not a mystery. Consciousness is not mysterious experientially, although we may have a mysterious experience.

Consciousness thrives on objects because they reflect consciousness back to itself. Sensory tissue is the ideal object as it draws attention to a primal source of consciousness. Quiet expansion is perfectly suited to this task. Expansion is an involuntary movement that enhances attention when we *are not doing*. *Doing* inhibits a clear, attentive pathway, while the involuntary movement of *not doing* feeds and sustains attention.

Attention can move between body and mind and then settles on itself. The beyondness experience begins with attention. We cannot *do* beyondness, but we can cultivate the attention that invites it. What begins as a local, focused attention disperses to become an ultimate unified experience.

> Be attentive to sensation and then immerse yourself into the nature and quality of attention itself. Highlight attention with the group. Examine the relationship between the quality of attention and the quality of consciousness. Refine attention until it opens into an expansive awareness as a group experience. Talk about it!

UNIFICATION

Being attentive to sensation teaches us how to be attentive to consciousness. Sensory attention directs us into personal consciousness. Attention to consciousness strengthens and intensifies consciousness. To shift consciousness we have to be attentive to and aware of consciousness.

Finite and infinite

Experience is finite. Our minds are unable to imagine galaxies without end extending out into infinity. The concept of infinity could not exist without the finite because we would have nothing to compare infinity to. We are finite and cannot imagine the endlessness of infinity. The finite, the definable, is our reality.

Infinity is a decondensation. In quantum terms it is nonmanifest. As we approach a less definitive way of being the density of experience decondenses. Although *we become less,* we cannot experience infinity because all experience is a condensation. As long as we have conscious experience which is a condensation, we can never actualize infinity. Anything beyond this is an unrecordable trance state with limited value (unless we value trance). It may be sufficient to refine the finite, or the definite, while acknowledging the idea of infinity.

As practice takes us out of ourselves, or takes the self out of us, infinity may hover as a possibility. Transcending thought and sensation brings us closer to a *feeling of* an infinite aspect of existence. Rupert Sheldrake writes: "There is no evidence to suggest that there are infinite numbers of unobserved Universes" (Sheldrake 2011). Expansion has its limitations.

Passing beyond the separative ego may be infinite enough in that it enables us to look at ourselves through a broader lens. We can move between the ego and spatial consciousness. We can slip between substance and emptiness, the known and the unknown, the finite and the projected infinite. The feeling of a *potential more* without direct proof of its existence gives us the sense of possibility. The feeling is enough.

Our tissue and our behavior have manifested out of something. Perhaps out of space, ether, gas, energy, an inaccessible presence, or a vaporous ground of being lying beyond and yet within us. The unmanifest may be a reality because we can conceive of it and in conceiving (conception) we give it life. This kind of speculation is based on experiences that arise during class work and is worthy of reference and discussion. It needs no conclusions. In any event, there are none. Inconclusion is a productive part of the process, if only to move us further beyond ourselves. We can say that we "saw something," in itself an understanding, and one that may loosen habitual behavior.

Tissue sense is a reference point for material reality. Body presence and density is the ideal basis from which we can venture into something less definitive. We remain finite as we pass through substance and move into a less finite experience. Dissolving conditioning blurs the margin between finite and what we might perceive as an infinite experience.

Chapter 10

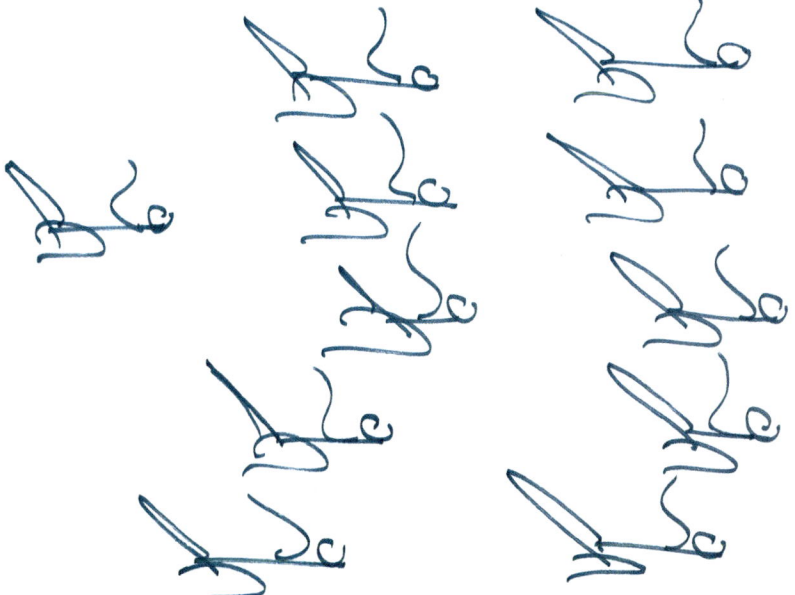

> Why does something have to be there? The feeling of a potential "more" gives extraordinary space to consciousness.

Confrontation

The habitual self relentlessly disturbs spatial consciousness. Investing in sensation does not guarantee avoiding excessive mental activity. We are continually confronted by conditioning. David Bohm put it succinctly:

The conditioning blocks us, because it creates a pressure to maintain what is familiar and old, and makes people frightened to consider anything new. So, reality is limited by the message which has already been deeply impressed on the brain cells from early child-hood. ... You adopt the idea that this block is truth because it relieves the pressure of uncertainty. (Bohm in Wilber 1982)

It is debatable how frightened we are to consider anything new. Our work focuses on breaking through the known to make new discoveries. Nevertheless, confronting an impasse of conditioned responses can stir an anxiety associated with the past. Strong sensations provoke conditioned reactions, but so might unifying sensations as we experience unaccustomed freedom.

Through no fault of our own we have embodied conditioned patterns from a past merging with the present. Psychotherapy confronts sometimes buried, and often painful, feelings. That mankind as a whole is conditioned has been suggested for centuries. Freud suggested that inner tensions were an inevitable consequence of instinctual drives pushing against social and cultural restrictions. Add

UNIFICATION

to this the tension of relationships, personal history, wants and not-wants, plus the tension provoked by the physical aspects of our work, and we have significant resistance. Everyone in the group may be confronted by themselves in some way.

Our work fulfills its scope by acknowledging the confrontational aspects of being conditioned. Conditioned reactions are magnified by sustained focus and give an opportunity for meaningful change. We can pass through ourselves time and again until the changes are more sustainable. In so doing we qualify to guide others through a similar experience. If students are unfamiliar with the depth of the process, we can apply additional presence to draw out trust.

You can see why choiceless practice arose. Choice risks a densification during an enlightened flow of decondensation. When conditioning reclaims its territory, we might choose to return to calmness, or sensation, or simply trust attention. When attention is at its most refined, adjustments take place spontaneously. Sensation and consciousness follow the positive route. Choiceless awareness does not disturb itself. Playing our sensory edges plays between rational and spatial consciousness and takes us beyond a compulsion to get it right.

The penetrant mind

One aspect of the mind is conditioned, another is unconditioned, and yet another is empty. The conundrum is that we get to the empty aspect by passing through the other two. We experience an egoless mind through the ego itself. The ego is the agent of subliminal consciousness, the mediator between the idea of depth and depth itself. Yoga masters understood that going into experiences dissolved the experiences. They passed through sensation, thought, and emotion and came out the other side into an emptiness they saw as freedom. We consciously acknowledge and penetrate turbulent patterns, so that consciousness may reorganize itself in an alternative light. The mind penetrates familiar sensation and thought like a laser. We arrive at emptiness.

> Penetrate thought and sensation with the part of your mind that does not register either. Leave thinking and feeling in the background of your experience. Observe *your* self pass through *your* self into emptiness. Teach from where you find yourself. Hold the reins while cutting them loose.

Some people appear to live transcendently unaffected by themselves or by life. The word *transcendent* implies moving beyond or above (something). It also means mystical, mystic, or ascendant. Mystical experience is an extension of everyday experience. It is a matter of degree. Many people have an awakened understanding beneath the surface but may not tune into it. Why would they if it has not occurred to them? We invite others to slip into a spatially unitive consciousness. Spatial consciousness comes forward. But transcendent experiences are also polarized. Nontranscended elements remain. Less finite experience expands from a definitive base.

Chapter 10

Mystical experience and creative insight spring from physical and mental sensation. Transcendence is a reality not that far removed from common experience.

Beyond thought

When thought moves to the background of our experience or leaves entirely, albeit for short periods, consciousness can find the space to reset itself, to shift.

Sense of self is not diminished by the absence of thought. Sense of self arises from and is enhanced by sensation and consciousness, as they come to the foreground of awareness.

Totality may be a thoughtless experience. Physicist David Bohm takes an interesting look at thought:

Almost all of mankind's thought is aimed at self-deception, which momentarily relieves pressures arising from this way of thinking, of being separate, and it produces pressures. When a person is under pressure any thought that comes in to relieve that pressure will be accepted as true. But immediately that leads to some more pressure because it's wrong and then you take another thought to relieve that thought. (Bohm in Wilber 1982)

Thought is not unitive because it is only a part of the whole of consciousness. Thought is either on the inside looking out or on the outside looking in. It separates itself from a unified whole. The word *reality* is based on the Latin word *res* meaning *matter* or *thing*. *Res* is a derivative of the word *rere* meaning *think*. Thoughts are *things* having substance that appear to be our reality. Thoughts can be our reality, and we become our thoughts. Physicist Renee Weber observed: "Thought is a fossilized kind of consciousness operating within the 'known' and thus by definition is uncreative" (Weber in Wilber 1982).

Some things cannot be understood by thinking. Thought cannot follow the inward movement of the mind. Thought is aware of its own nature but cannot think itself out of thinking. Following mental behavior may invite a self-reflection and introspection that weighs itself down.

Thought is transcended to some degree by being attentive to it. The mind can watch its content but we can disperse thought by entering into the *fact* of thought without referring to its content. This is an advanced strategy demanding an intense practice. But we can use the ever-present reality of sensation to take us beyond thought. Focused attention on sensation begins to dissolve thought.

Beyond sensation

Sensation gives a material focus that leads us into spatial consciousness. We cannot go beyond sensation because we *are* sensation. Sensory nerves are operative whether or not we pay attention to what we are feeling. But we can go beyond the significance that we give to sensation. When we enter a house for the first time we do not linger at the doorway. We pass through to find out what lies within, to explore its unknown space.

We can leave sensation in the background of awareness and gently return to it when we are distracted by thought. When we have finished with the sensations of the breath, the contact with the ground, the expansion

UNIFICATION

of the superficial tissue, we can come back to deep, seemingly infinite stillness. This is where consciousness can reset itself.

Many traditional practitioners viewed bodywork as an ego-driven self-examination unsuitable for spiritual realization. But as much as we refine sensation, it is always there, telling us we are present, that we exist. Experience is a sensation. Meditation draws attention to sensation, and sensation is an ideal meditation. We cannot transcend sensation entirely and would not want to as it provides the anchor from which we can venture into unknown territory. Sensation gives the mind a point of entry into a deeper consciousness.

We can transcend and refine gross sensation into a more subtle experience. But how subtle is subtle? We can refine the relationship between the ego and sensation until sensation becomes the predominant feature. The fragmentation of the ego, its tendency to move from one thing to the next and back again, can be addressed by sensing the skin as one piece. The awakening and unification of surface sensation unifies the ego, a necessary requirement if we are to move beyond our familiar selves. If we are to transcend ego dominance the ego must be integrated and it must be healthy.

Sensation is the key but we might use it as a spiritual aphrodisiac that loses potency when the practice is over. Reliance on sensation alone has its limitations. Attention can magnify and then dissolve sensation. Foreground sensations disperse into the background as the next sensation arrives to be transcended: an ongoing experience inviting us to pass through ever-present sensory activity.

The tantric approach celebrates sensation while transcending it. The Sanskrit word *tantra* comes from the root *tan* meaning to *expand or continue*. According to one definition *tantra is that which expands knowledge*. The *knowledge* is not factual information. Georg Feuerstein observed: "Tantrism is a means of acquiring direct knowledge of the oneness of all existence" (Feuerstein 1992).

Tantric practices refine and pass through sensation into expansion. Material expansion leading into nonmaterial expansion is one sensation. Sensory exploration can provide a lifetime of enriching work, and new sensations provide a bedrock of inspiration. At some point we can refine our relationship to sensation and transcend excessive identification with the body. We can follow where sensory intelligence leads and enter aspects of consciousness that hold deeper transformative shifts.

We can overthink and overdescribe sensation. Sensory descriptions are filtered through conditioned thought. Describing sensation to oneself and to others is essential, but, once described, sensation should be left to its own intelligence. By the time we have described the sensation it may have moved on. Excessive description inhibits sensations that need to roam. Transformation occurs by refining our relationship to sensation.

Consciousness thrives in the space between sensation and its acknowledgment. Attention to sensation without descriptive thought holds us in the present. The thought *I am feeling the superficial fascia* might be appropriate but is limited by its recognition. Our potential is more profound than sensory satisfaction. Consciousness functioning in the present is free from recognition.

Chapter 10

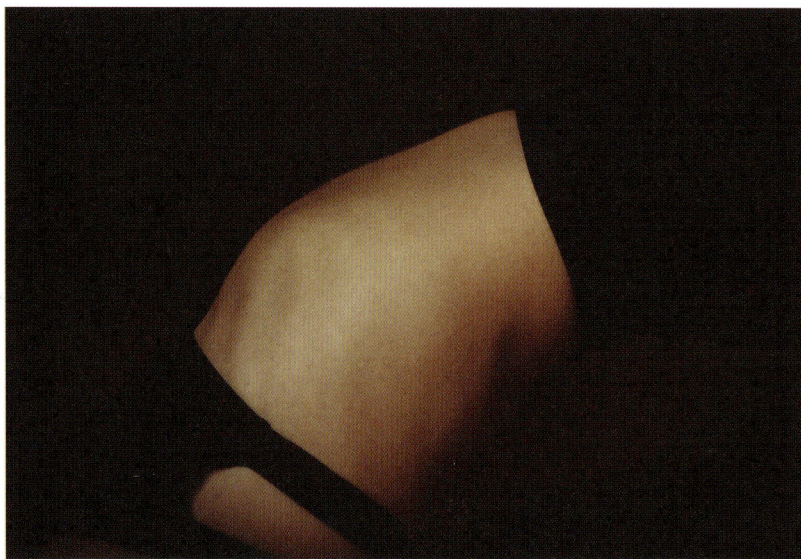

Consciousness thrives in the space between sensation and its acknowledgment.

Sensation is finite but consciousness has broader possibilities. Passing through feelings of finiteness gives the *impression* of entering infiniteness. Focused attention to sensation shifts consciousness. We can then address consciousness directly as it moves beyond its limitations. In turn, excursions into the further reaches of consciousness change the body. The energy of consciousness devoid of thought transforms tissue. Tissue becomes lighter, softer, and more expansive when freed from the imposition of thought. The relationship between sensation and consciousness is an ongoing process of refinement. Penetrative consciousness disperses sensation to become the sensation of spatial and then dynamic consciousness.

We are, at once, sensory technicians and agents of an alternative consciousness. There is more potential depth in consciousness than can be found in the material body. Consciousness expands beyond the physical sensation of expansion.

We may drift between sensation, thought, and varying intensities of consciousness. But dynamic consciousness will out. Acknowledging dynamic consciousness strengthens its potential for transformation.

Detaching, witnessing, and waiting

Transcending mental and sensory activity requires a measured detachment. When we are attached to our experience we cannot pass through it.

Traditional practitioners took nonattachment to extremes. They viewed attachment of any kind as the antithesis of totality. We may be more selective. It might be enough for some just to take the edge off, while others may wish to take it further. Jean Gebser understood that some form of detachment was needed for personal growth. He wrote: "There is a need for a certain detachment toward oneself and the world, a gradually maturing equilibrium of all

Unification

the inherent components and consciousness structures predisposed in ourselves, in order that we may prepare the basis for the leap into the new mutation" (Gebser 1949/1985).

We cannot just be "unattached." Life thrives on attachment. But less attachment in some areas may be productive, as it frees us for a broader perspective and helps us realize what we are attached to and why we are attached to it. Beyond the visceral bonds between us, the common sense of financial security, and personal creativity some of our attachments and the degree to which they hold us may be an aspect of our conditioning.

However, within the process that we find ourselves in, it is natural for students and teachers to form an attachment. The yoga tradition saw fit for a student to attach himself to a teacher in preparation for a reliance on his own experience. Teacher–student bonding enhances the process of learning. It is normal and desirable for oxytocin release to bond groups. Teachers are attached to their students, to their teaching, and to the stimulation of new discoveries. Healthy attachment is not an emotional need but respects the space between us and invites more relaxation, simplicity, clarity, and receptivity. A soft, quiet *detached attachment* opens the group field.

The yoga experience flourishes in response to a detached focus. We can be deeply attentive to the skin, the mind, and the sense of self without the attachment that closes consciousness. We can be simultaneously attentive to and removed from ourselves. Standing back gives space for unpredictable changes. We see more clearly from a distance.

We can move more deeply by cultivating our witness. Our witness has been familiar since childhood. Witnessing our internal behavior is the essential aspect of conscience, of understanding ourselves, and is the foundation of intelligent relationship. We witness thought, analysis, emotion, reaction, and response. Witnessing provides the space within which experience can change itself. We can witness resistance, engagement, and expansion. Witnessing renders experience less personal and therefore less conditioned.

Practicing light detachment and witnessing teaches us how to *wait* for the involuntary spread of tissue and for consciousness to clear. *Waiting* refines sensation and frees dynamic consciousness for action. Courting sensitivity by waiting draws attention to the fact that movements and moments are never the same. Gross movements and mental attitudes may appear the same but on the essential level finer sensations and mental states are fluid and they move. We can wait for the ongoing reorganization of tissue and emotion to teach us about our impatience and conditioned reactions. Waiting and listening are inseparable.

Waiting underpins an ancient philosophy and more often than not eliminates the need for action. In this respect there is no such thing as repetition. You cannot repeat an existent flow of spontaneous involuntary activity.

In quantum and yogic terms, experience, however subtle, has substance. All experiences are condensations. The experience of dissolving an experience is the next experience to be dissolved, until we find ourselves in a twilight realm of vast expansion without

Chapter 10

content. Our witness remains to record the experience. When attention is infused with detachment and waiting, we detect the slightest shift in consciousness, spotlight the smallest anticipation, and enable the impulse to do or describe pass by.

> Detach yourself from all aspects of your experience. Witness all the sensory comings and goings and fluctuations of mental activity. As spatial consciousness arrives wait for all activity to transpire and disperse. Communicate your experience to the group. Guide and support them from a profound space.

The force of consciousness

The primal stages of an awakening consciousness would have been an involuntary process. We would not have *decided* to *be* consciously aware. Our conscious will would have developed at a later stage on the back of an archaic consciousness. Consciousness is involuntary. We do not have to think about remaining consciously aware, but we are aware of our consciousness. Conscious awareness can look at the fact of consciousness. We can, through the ego, apply conscious awareness to consciousness which in turn can reveal the force of its involuntary nature. "Strength or intensity of consciousness cannot be brought to consciousness by thinking alone since thinking knows only spatial sequentiality" (Gebser 1949/1985).

For our purpose consciousness has two possibilities. It can spread with surface sensation enabling the ego to take a broader view, and it can also be incisive, cutting through all unnecessary activity. An incisive consciousness emerges to penetrate ego consciousness from within. Consciousness penetrates itself as it penetrates thought and sensation. We can experience the *texture* of consciousness. Sensation provides the base until consciousness becomes its own stabilizing force.

Consciousness becomes the predominant sensation by awakening its own dullness. Consciousness is a sense and a sensation. We feel consciously aware and feel consciousness. Sensation becomes consciousness and consciousness becomes sensation. Consciousness is a felt sense. We can feel consciousness *knowing* and acting upon itself.

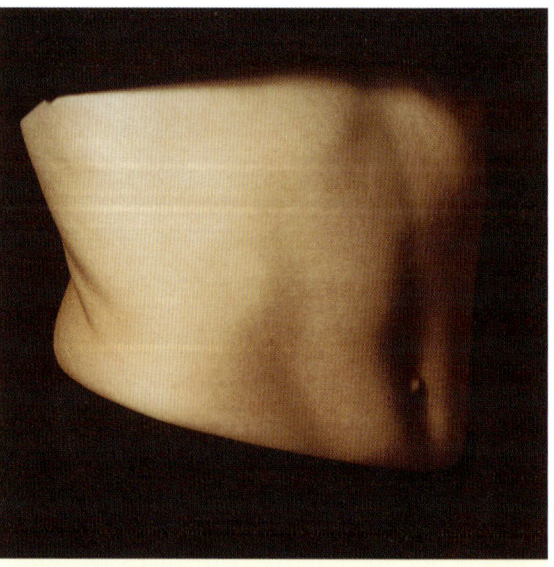

Sensation becomes consciousness and consciousness becomes sensation. Consciousness is a felt sense. We can feel consciousness knowing and acting on itself.

UNIFICATION

The force of consciousness draws us into a seemingly endless and lucid space. A pure sense of self flows from a tide of immutable consciousness. Consciousness meets itself. An unobstructed view of consciousness draws attention to its *intensity*. Pure vibrant consciousness can be experienced as an all-encompassing emotive force. All other emotional content is dissolved by a tide of wakeful consciousness.

Dynamic consciousness does not think and cannot be summoned by thought. Its unsullied force dissolves habitual reflection and experience. Its power sustains the space from which profound insight materializes. Power yoga concerns dynamic consciousness, is beyond anything we can construct, and inhabits a realm of its own. The ego has the idea of exploring the further reaches of consciousness but having made contact is blown apart by its discovery. Dynamic consciousness can be seen and experienced as the nucleus of everything that we mean by the term consciousness. Dynamic consciousness is nuclear. It evaporates everything in its path.

For consciousness to penetrate itself it must feel and know itself in every moment. This demands unwavering attention and a piercing interest in breaking down the energy invested in maintaining our conditioned state.

> Consider consciousness as a sensation. Pierce all of your sensory and mental activity by using the sensation of consciousness. Consciousness becomes its own penetrative tool. It blows away all other activity.

Consciousness is normally perceived as an abstraction because its underlying nature is hidden by ongoing content. We cannot see the wood for the trees. When consciousness is freed from content we can experience its texture. As with surrounding space, consciousness has substance. Quantum theory and yoga suggest that consciousness is subtle matter connecting all mankind. The sensation of consciousness densifies within, between, and around us. "Each individual manifests the consciousness of mankind" (Bohm in Wilber 1982).

There may be one unitive consciousness: a proposal made by many enlightened thinkers and one that may resonate with our own experience. Consciousness studies itself. Krishnamacharya explained to his son Desikachar that pure consciousness may be short-lived: "My father used to say that we need a lot of effort for a moment of yogic experience. It is not possible to stay continuously in the state where consciousness is master for long. But that one moment is worth trying for, because we discover something: a very special joy" (Desikachar & Krusche 2014).

There are intensities of joy. A joyful experience may last for more than a moment or so, as demonstrated by the spontaneous irrepressible smile, the *grin of knowing*. Joyful experiences loosen the conditioned mind. Consciousness knows a good thing when it sees it. Habitual experience assimilates the effects of the sustainable moments of dynamic consciousness with the potential for changing our behavior, our timing, and our communicability in relationship.

Chapter 10

The void

Passing through thought and sensation gains access to the proverbial void, an experience of infinite inner depth and emptiness. The word *void* has various definitions that include: nothingness, space, abyss, without content, unoccupied, and desolate. We might encounter this unblemished, uninhabited, desolate consciousness. Yoga might refer to this phenomenon as the core of universal being within ourselves, a space from which all realization emanates.

The void experience touches on an abyss of nothingness, as if we are organized around a seemingly infinite space where thought and ideas cannot survive, where experience itself is atomized. We might sense a fine inner margin between the material self and an inner infinity. This margin cannot be totally crossed, and we cannot enter the void completely. To do so would be to disappear, an experience of no experience, recorded by Eastern adepts as the pinnacle of transcendent yoga. We can, however, hover at the void's edge and peer into it.

The ego must be grounded in dynamic consciousness and light physical sensation in order to observe an inner void from a place of material reality. We become inner-space travellers without abandoning ship, suspended at the edge of another reality, observing inner vastness on a universal scale. Depending on the stability of our witness the void may be hospitable or otherwise. We might experience an unoccupied space filled with *knowing* or a barren and pointless mindscape.

Penny, a student in her seventies, recounted her experience during a class:

> "When I was in my early twenties, I was taking LSD. Went on a trip where I didn't have any visual hallucinations but took away the layers of my superficiality to try and find myself. I came to a black hole and nearly fell in. I remember screaming and tangling up the layers again so I could go on existing. On Tuesday I came to the hole again, looked in and it was fine. This round trip has taken me about 50 years. The experience was profound!"

Transcending ourselves is not necessarily reflected by a void experience. Emptiness has no interest in itself. The void is a transformative yet temporary adventure of consciousness. If and when it happens it indicates a more total dissolution of the familiar self at the time.

Trips

Within a few hours one small pill can achieve what normally takes years of meditation and yoga. Deeper yoga experiences are often compared to LSD experiences. Both experiences magnify consciousness and a sense of oneness with all things. B. K. S. Iyengar commented that, from what he had heard about LSD, he frequently had these experiences during his practices. Alan Watts, philosopher and Zen Buddhist, described in detail his LSD experiences. R. D. Laing used LSD in therapy sessions. Obstetrician Michel Odent suggested that women giving birth came close to the LSD experience, and yoga scholar Georg Feuerstein acknowledged LSD

Unification

as a spiritual short cut. Michael Pollan's book *How To Change Your Mind* explores the parallels between meditation and LSD and the newly found benefits of small amounts of LSD in regard to mental health (Pollan 2018).

Neuroscientist Antonio Damasio suggests that consciousness pulsates in a wavelike fashion. I experienced this in the mid-1970s during an LSD experience while practicing yoga. I also felt a pulsation and wavelike movement of the atmosphere surrounding my body. It is known that gravity comes in waves and that space is filled with energy. Recent yoga experiences (without the LSD) suggest a waveless movement of existence, a constant flowing outward from an inner space, an experience also recorded by LSD experimenters. Perhaps waves and particles of existence, as suggested by physics, lie within the waveless experience. Conversely, wavelessness may exist beneath waves and particles!

Feelings of expanded consciousness induced by LSD suggest that normal consciousness is habitually contracted. Michael Pollan refers to the meditation studies conducted by neuroscientist Judson Brewer. Brewer found that a felt sense of consciousness expansion correlates with a drop in the activity of an area of the cortical brain associated with self-referential processing (Pollan 2018). Self-reference, although essential for understanding and processing one's experience, can strengthen the "I" beyond intelligent levels through incessant repetition. Consciousness expansion reduces the contractive sense of *I am*.

Pollan describes a sense of consciousness expansion during the days following psychedelic experiences. As his ego dominance reduced, Pollan noted a reduction in the attention he paid to the past and future. He became more present. He also became aware of a sense of *consciousness contraction* when feeling fearful, defensive, or worried. His experimentation revealed a quality of consciousness ranging between expansion and contraction, which is an experience that is at least available to us, if not commonplace. We may have this experience on a daily basis once attuned to the nature of consciousness. For millennia various cultures have ingested hallucinogenic substances in combination with practices that open consciousness to intense spiritual experiences. The value of LSD in this regard is debatable. There is a difference between the immediate short-term effects of psychedelic drugs and the benefits of a consistent practice over time.

Noticing the contraction of consciousness presents an opportunity to restore its expansion, a trick of the mind, and is a realization that can be imparted in class work.

No one knows

Along with consciousness and experience, the source of all things remains unknown. Consciousness, experience, and the ground of existence are united by their mysterious origin. Mysticism and physics ponder over what consciousness actually is, how we experience it, and how we connect to one another or to a grand scheme of things. An unknown basis for profound experience gives space for elaborate possibilities.

Science studies the unknown and mystics may live by it. We simply engage with it. Ken Wilber writes:

Chapter 10

The work of these scientists … is too important to be weighed down with wild speculations on mysticism. And mysticism itself is too profound to be hitched to phases of scientific theorizing. Let them appreciate each other, and let their dialogue and mutual exchange of ideas never cease. But unwarranted and premature marriages usually end in divorce and all too often a divorce that terribly damages both parties. (Wilber 1982)

New physics is far from a consensus as to the nature of subatomic reality.

Ken Wilber does acknowledge that mysticism and physics are agreed that everything is connected (something that may seem obvious to the uncomplicated awareness of childhood). He notes that for the physicist *oneness* implies an all-encompassing fabric of subatomic particles, but for the mystic *oneness* implies everything is simply one. Both views are not that far apart, in that mystical or yogic practices produce vibrational and spatial sensations that suggest oneness with everything. We often feel the inseparability of body, psyche, and totality. Physicist David Bohm proposed that the mystic is someone who has had direct experience of the mystery of a reality which transcends the possibility of description.

We can and do find ourselves guiding others toward an indescribable experience and in so doing acknowledge its indescribableness.

Many are of the opinion that should an unknown reveal itself it would do so from within us. The unknown resides within us.

William James saw cosmic realization as an aspect of a hidden mind. He wrote:

Total reactions are different from casual reactions, and total attitudes are different from usual attitudes. To get at them you must go behind the foreground of existence and reach down to that curious sense of the whole residual cosmos as an everlasting presence, intimate or alien, terrible or amusing, lovable or odious, which in some degree everyone possesses. (James 1902/2018).

Bohm emphasized the importance for physics, biology, and psychology for what he called "formative causation," i.e., "an ordered and structured inner movement that is essential to what things are." In the ancient view "the notion of formative cause was considered to be essentially of the same nature for the mind as it was for life and for the cosmos as a whole" (Bohm in Wilber 1982). Consciousness is seen as an aspect of the cosmos and continuous with it.

Quantum physics is generally based on assumptions that cannot be proved and at best are probabilities arising out of possibilities. "Theoretical science is not primarily concerned with observing things but observing ideas … an idea is an instrument for grasping a broader reality … you can't suddenly inject consciousness variables into physics" (Bohm in Wilber 1982). Science is interested in mystical experience but can neither validate or invalidate it. Mystical experience cannot be proved (nor can the movement of ordinary experience). It thrives on possibilities beyond proof. Proof would see the end of it, and there would be no unknown, no mystery or mysticism. Science in this regard is the

Unification

ego's attempt to understand itself in relation to the nature of existence. Science may prove unhelpful in understanding the ego's dispersion into the bigger picture because science is an extension of the ego and therefore reinforces the ego.

Physicist Renee Weber asked Bohm about his characterization of the state of physics (at the time). He comments: "they [the physicists] use the idea of fields and particles but when you press them they have no image whatsoever what these things are, and they have no content other than the results of what they can calculate with their equations … We are trying to give a description of reality whether wrong or right" (Bohm in Wilber 1982).

Unification defies scientific inquiry because the totality of everything contains science within it. Science is a product of totality and as such is not in a position to understand it, or discover its source. The experience of vastness encompasses science. It can certainly *feel* as if a larger field is at work, and some areas of science show that a subtle form of communication exists, but it is just not known how.

Rupert Sheldrake recognizes the limitations of science. He writes:

We may of course, simply regard the origin of the Universe and the creativity within it as an impenetrable mystery and leave it at that. If we choose to look further, we find ourselves in the presence of several long-established traditions of thought about the ultimate creative source, whether this is conceived of as the One, Brahma, the Void, the Tao, the eternal embrace of Shiva and Shakti, or the Holy Trinity. In all of these traditions, we sooner or later arrive at the limits of conceptual thought, and also at a recognition of these limits. Only mystical insight, contemplation or enlightenment can take us beyond them. (Sheldrake 2011)

Science proposes a quantumness of consciousness but cannot say what consciousness is. Scientists sought clarity from the subjective experience of Eastern practitioners who went into themselves to arrive at the conclusions that science seeks. Eastern philosophy arose out of personal experience in the absence of scientific evidence. The experience was given as absolute. Knowledge was based on acknowledgment without explanation.

Modern physics is a supportive science but difficult to grasp. Its proposals are often beyond experience because they are formulated by mathematical equations that frequently change as they are realized. We end up with the idea and not the experience.

The subjective experience of less density, the absence of distinctive thought, an uncluttered consciousness, and a spatial connection to beyondness draw us into a transcendent field, as documented by the yoga masters, and can give us a lifetime of ongoing inquiry and speculation. Their philosophy arose from the realization that explanations are fixed, have no movement, and therefore no possibility.

Rupert Sheldrake writes: "Science lacks subjective values, we may be guided by science in order to make life more livable, but the subjective experience of life has qualities that are outside the domain of science" (Sheldrake 2011).

Chapter 10

Amit Goswami, author of *The Self-Aware Universe*, asks: "If consciousness is the fabric of the world, how do we find new laboratory experiments to confirm the idea? This is one of the remaining questions" (Goswami 1995).

Wisdom is not the domain of the physicist. We are more likely to seek wisdom from the mystic, but physicists such as Bohm exhibited deep insight. When proven, some things lose their potential. When the mystery goes, we move on. What becomes known leads on to the next unknown. Speculation and unknowing give unlimited space for the creation of personal insight and understanding. Science is a tool for objective understanding, not an experience. We cannot live moment to moment by science. Sheldrake proposes that scientific theories are, like myths, mental constructs attempting to make sense of the world. *Lucid noticing*, regardless of the outcome is *our* science. Group work, its field, produces a heightened sensitivity to a shared totality.

Universal experience

The immeasurability of the universal experience is not proof that it does not exist and makes it all the more compelling. Existence is unquantifiable. Without knowing a universe existed, we might still have a sense of infinity, although limited because human imagination cannot imagine something that does not end somewhere. We may return to a one-with-everything sensation based on intrauterine experience, prior to ego development. We may be returning to a spatial feeling following conception: the space-traveling blastosphere.

As we lighten and decondense, we may project our sense of freedom from ourselves onto an out-there possibility. It may be easier to find solace in a universal consciousness than to trust an unknown aspect of our deeper selves.

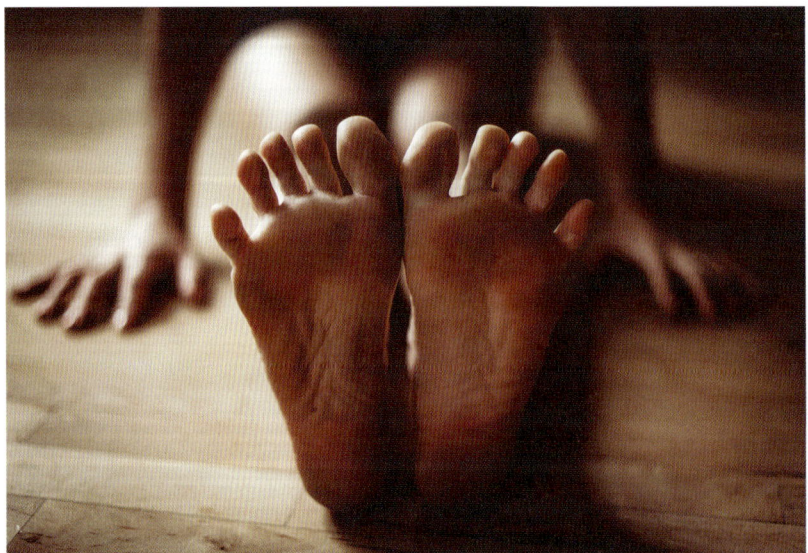

Lucid noticing is our science. Group work produces a heightened sensitivity to a shared totality.

Unification

It is a fact (of physics) that we are a condensation of energy manifesting as animate matter. We connect and communicate through space. We blend with one another and with a local and nonlocal field. We are the souls of space, a unified field of energies blending with cosmic energy. Sense of self flows outward from an unidentifiable inner source that has no center.

Perhaps we rekindle magical or mythical consciousness beginning with a heightened sensitivity to the space around us and an inexplicable sense of wonder and amazement.

Speculation informs teaching and gives space for creativity. It is tempting to fill emptiness with conceptual possibilities. The "something larger" experience fits perfectly. Profound insight arises out of the void. As our inner world empties, we feel continuous with our outer world. We may simply be in touch with our subconscious. Krishnamurti, one of the most sensitive teachers in his field, made no reference to cosmic intelligence. He may have thought that addressing the conditioned mind was enough to get on with.

Universal sensation

The ultimate unifying experience is the direct physical sense of feeling continuous with a universal fabric. It is a sensation, it has texture, and it begins with the body. Giving complete focused attention to an area of tissue opens awareness to a sense of totality beyond the idea of totality. We experience a combined sensory awakening of tissue and consciousness leading to a focus on consciousness as a universal field. For example, surface tissue spreading at the back of the waist gives a sense of self-expansion outward beyond the body. Profound local sensations of lightness and space take consciousness into the space beyond.

Iyengar, like many before him, was unequivocal regarding the relationship between physical and cosmic experience. Divinity revealed itself to Iyengar through his body: "Cosmic intelligence is the organizing system of the Universe" (Iyengar 2005). Universal feelings emerge as a consequence of significant shifts in tension.

> Be attentive to the tissue around your waist and chest. Apply the lightest engagement. Sense a radiation spread in all directions throughout your whole body. Have no waist or chest. Sense the skin of your entire body spread and dissolve into the space around you. Feel a universal connectivity. Feel inseparable from universal space. Share the experience with those occupying the space around you.

A private universe

As far out as things may get, unification begins as a private experience. For William James, the cosmic experience was an awakening of our subliminal consciousness combined with our awareness that there is a cosmos. The *idea* of universal consciousness arises from knowing a universe exists. The *feeling* of a cosmic consciousness may arise from the fact that we are conscious of the cosmos. We include our knowledge of its existence in our expansive experience.

Chapter 10

The universe is an observable fact said to extend beyond itself into infinite space. Most people have a universal awareness. But the enhanced universal experience is one of subjective physical unity. The cosmic experience emerges as the ego dissolves. Alexander Lowen suggested that "the ego differentiates itself out of the id only to lose itself in the id in life's supreme moments" (Lowen 1958). (The *id* was the term used by Freud to denote the primitive part of the personality, our driving force residing in the unconscious.)

The mind is a private kaleidoscope of memories, expectations, evaluations, ideas, thoughts, and feelings, plus a myriad of shadowy background activity. The sum total of this activity is grounded in consciousness and influences its quality. We should acknowledge the content and complexity of each mind as we invite others to enter their inner space. Damasio comments on individual consciousness: "Consciousness is a part of your mental process rather than external to it. Individual perspective, individual ownership of thought, and individual agency are the critical riches that core consciousness contributes to the mental process now unfolding in your organism" (Damasio 2000).

As activity disperses the resultant space gives a sense of vastness combined with an intensification of consciousness. Consciousness is freed from its confinement.

We may feel unified with the whole but the whole may be within us. Modern physics approaches this question holographically. A holograph looks at the relationship between the whole of something and its parts, suggesting that each part contains an image of the whole. Its totality is found in each of its components. The holographic theory suggests that the universe represents itself within each of us. As each cell contains information of the whole body, each brain contains a holographic representation of the universe. We may touch on a universal space within us as we peer into our void. Such a possibility may arise and be magnified in each person as a group engages in a unitive practice. A primal field may transmit a holographic resonance received by each one of us, an experience recorded by yoga practitioners and mystics in their own terms throughout the ages.

Is the universe aware of itself?

Further to this is a sense that the universe *has* consciousness, the ultimate projection. Or is it? If a universal consciousness exists perhaps our experience is the tool it uses to reveal itself. Personal and group experiences may be expressions of cosmic intelligence. Might the universe be aware of itself? A gentle stretch of the imagination is not beyond traditional beliefs. Dr Amit Goswami, professor of physics at the Institute for Theoretical Sciences at the University of Oregon, in his compelling book *The Self-Aware Universe*, draws on a synthesis of modern physics and spirituality. Blending scientific theory with the recorded experience of yoga and meditation practitioners through the ages, Goswami eloquently proposes that consciousness is the foundation for all creation, theorizing that we have evolved out of a grand consciousness aware of itself. Factual

UNIFICATION

or not, the supposition may bring comfort to some. If we think we feel the presence of an infinite intelligence, then why shouldn't we believe in it? This belief, in one form or another, has brought solace and hope to mankind throughout time.

Dr Goswami points to the subjective experimentation and experience of the individual and the necessity for meditation and yoga. Toward the end of his thesis he writes: "The fundamental unverifiable (in the scientific sense) idealist metaphysic is a one-liner: Consciousness is the ground of all being and our self-consciousness is That consciousness" (Goswami 1995). In contrast, William James commented:

In the religious life the control is felt as "higher"; but it is primarily the higher faculties of our own hidden mind which are controlling, the sense of union with the power beyond us is a sense of something, not merely apparently, but literally true. … Yet it is only a doorway, and difficulties present themselves as soon as we step through it, and ask how far our transmarginal consciousness carries us if we follow it on its remoter side. Here the over-beliefs begin … and tell us that the finite self rejoins the absolute self, for it was always one with God and identical with the soul of the world. (James 1902/2018)

The perception of a self-aware universe might include the idea of its awareness of us. Is God watching (over) us or do we touch on an innocent, archaic, mythical, or magical consciousness? Our in-the-moment heightened sensory experiences reveal the extraordinary capacity for consciousness to deepen, intensify, and project itself. Consciousness presents us with an open canvas on which to paint possibilities that may or may not be founded in reality. Our experience based on our senses is *our* reality. Our imagination, as a sense, is an extension of this reality, giving us food for thought, debate, and the potential for group discussion.

Being centerless

Dissolving physical density evokes a centerless feeling of inner space and emptiness. This feeling is beyond the well-documented tensegrity experience whereby bones acting as spacers push outward from the center of the body. Centerlessness indicates a total release of tension within and throughout the area between the pelvis and thorax as if all tissues dissolve. The feeling of a spatial center enables a fluidity of perception and spirit. Space is the ideal element for merging with totality. Physical space, like the mind, can go everywhere and anywhere. Emptiness (the most extreme lightness) comes from opening the skin and surface tissue, sensing into and beyond the depth of the spine and deep tissue, and by passing through all emotional and mental activity as it passes through us.

Consciousness penetrates and refines sensation into a feeling of space. Emptiness, the sense of being here and not being here, gives a sense of infinite connectivity.

The sense of spatial consciousness and the sense of infinite space inform each other.

Chapter 10

Physicist Weber posits to physicist David Bohm: "If one had an experience of the limitless infinitude of space, one would have an infinitude of consciousness?" Bohm replies:

It would be consciousness which was infinite not in terms of extension but in its self-determined character. ... you could say that the infinity of being can map onto knowing, and thus knowing and being are ultimately identical in that infinity is not extensive but "intensive" ... that kind of being requires a space which is entirely different from that in which we display mechanical objects ... we could say that consciousness has to become commensurate with that different space in order to discover it. Consciousness in fact has to change its very state. (Weber and Bohm in Wilber 1982)

Here lies the potential of our work! The unification of spatial physical experience and spatial consciousness produces an intensification of consciousness or *dynamic consciousness*. Bohm also acknowledges the sense of *knowing,* as referred to elsewhere in this book.

Spatial sensation is the route to dynamic consciousness. We feel *centerless* as sensory nerves awaken to lightness and space. Physical space is synonymous with mind space and dissolves thought, self-reference, and conditioning. Dispersing density invites a sensory union with beyondness. Whether or not beyondness has intelligence is up for debate.

True depth has no anatomical or ego center: it is not a *place*, but simply the presence of space. Our deepest place is nonmaterial. We might experience a *stable vulnerability*. There is no structure to defend. We are detached because there is nothing to be attached to! When the center is free, conditioning loses its anchor and has no roots. Potential darkness within the void is countered by an outward flow of light. Self-consciousness and sensation empty as one movement as we become continuous with space. The energy that would be thought, description, or recognition flows through us. There is nothing to hold, simply an absence of materialization and condensation.

> This kind of experience requires the group to be in a seated position and should be conveyed with particular sensitivity and a grounded, generous sense of self. We should be clear on where we are going and the fact that the group is in a heightened state of awareness. We should return from this experience by keeping the eyes down and waiting before the group reconnects locally with us and with one another.

Each point of reference is a self-reference because we refer to our own experience of that referred to. The words "space" and "center," are not the experience, they have no movement within consciousness. One superfluous thought or word can impede the flow of knowing. We need wording that complements rather than inhibits the process of insight. This can only come from our own insight at the time of its arrival, and even then requires delicate consideration.

Unification

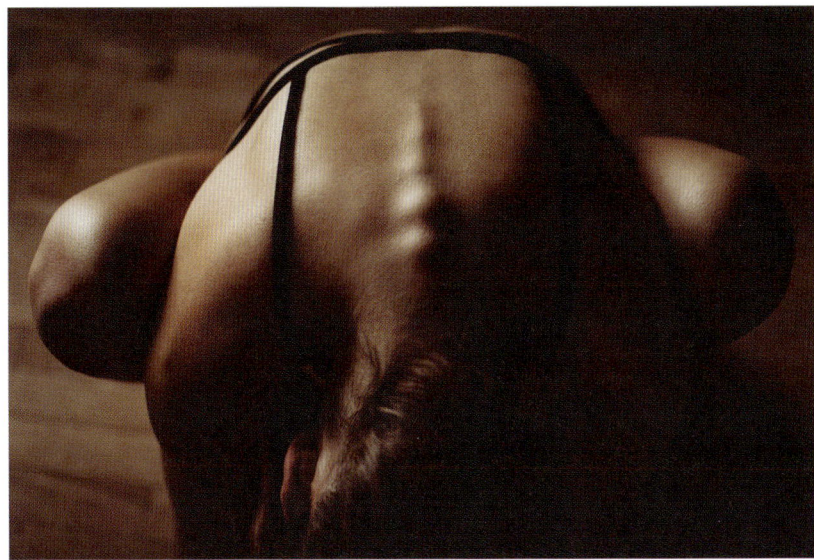

True depth has no anatomical or ego center: it is not a place, but simply the presence of space. Our deepest place is nonmaterial.

Transmitting, channeling, and downloading

We might feel that we *channel* from another time and place. Perhaps we tune into a morphic field from the past. Others may speak through us. Sheldrake writes:

When an organized system dies ... its organizing field disappears from that place. But in another sense, morphic fields do not disappear: they are potential organizing patterns of influence, and can appear again physically in other times and places, wherever the physical conditions are appropriate. When they do, so they contain within themselves a memory of their previous physical existences. (Sheldrake 2011)

Some teachers are particularly sensitive. Their words and insights may be influenced by a collective field beyond the current presence of group consciousness. Sheldrake's following proposal is compelling, suggesting that the more people that are involved, the greater the probability of a morphic resonance across time. Are we channeling a transcendent experience, realized over centuries by those who investigated their potential for transforming consciousness?

The process by which the past becomes present within morphic fields is called morphic resonance ... Morphic resonance plays a major part in cultural inheritance and sheds a new light on religious practices such as rituals and the use of mantras ... Morphic fields arise and evolve in time and space, and are influenced by what has actually happened ... By morphic resonance, structures of thought and experience that were common to many people in the past contribute to morphic fields. These fields contain as it were the average forms of previous experience defined in terms of probability. (Sheldrake 2011)

Chapter 10

Perhaps we download, channel, and transmit ways of being that have for centuries signified transformative experiences.

Perspective

The fact of materiality and nonmateriality is not the issue. It is how we perceive them. Material and nonmaterial engagement are interpenetrative and cross-refer. The tension of thought and the tension of sensation pass into and through each other. Presence, consciousness, memory, ideas, sensations, and emotions are tensions. Tension underlies experience and all experience is tension. Groups are united by the tension of sensation and consciousness. We connect through the gently powerful tension of expansion and *knowing*. Although physical expansion informs our presence it remains the lower rung on a ladder to something infinitely larger. Consciousness is an infinite feeling arising from sensation. The texture of consciousness provides an unsurpassable feeling of *being here and being out there*.

To whatever extent an experience may be enlightening, the quality of our relationship to the experience determines the quality of the transformation. The relationship between heightened sensation and intensive consciousness is put into perspective by acknowledging space around and within the entire experience. The intensity of consciousness and its sensory backdrop is supported by the coexistence of space. The fundamental principle supporting mystical insight is our investment in space. Giving space to and for our experience provides fertility for the birth of authentic insight.

Space and knowing

Investment in an ongoing spatial perspective brings us back to the expressive, almost haunting sense of knowing. William Braud, one of Lynne McTaggart's physicists, had read the Vedas, India's religious texts of the ancient Hindus, which described *siddhis* (psychic events) that would occur during profound meditative states. "The subject enters a state of unity with the single object being focused upon. In the highest state, the mediator experiences feelings of a type of omniscient knowing, a sense of seeing everywhere at once" (Braud in McTaggart 2003).

McTaggart refers to research showing that the brains of children under the age of five function permanently in alpha mode, the state of altered consciousness in adults, as opposed to the beta mode of ordinary mature consciousness. Children appear to be far more in touch with the *field* than the average adult: "In effect a child walks around in a state of permanent hallucination" (McTaggart 2003). We have had this experience as children – a lucid sense of *knowing* free from the impediment of knowledge and past experience.

The sense of knowing is familiar. Consciousness derives from the Latin words *scire* (to know) and *cum* (with). Consciousness is *to know with*. It also means *the sense of having perception*. The shared experience of a group *knows* and *perceives*. Knowing consciousness blending with the perception of inner and surrounding space indicates that we tap into something usually dulled to awareness. A sense of *knowing* nothing in particular implies that consciousness is free from the past and free

Unification

from speculation. *Knowing* runs parallel to the feeling that we *are*. We obviously *are*, but *knowing* draws from an intensified sense of *being*. Damasio describes "the unvarnished sense of self of our individual organism in the act of knowing." Further to this is the sense of a shared *knowing* of a group, providing the space within which insight can thrive.

There is a kind of knowing which penetrates to the very core of the universe, which offers truth as something at once beatific and comforting, and presents the human mind as being cradled in a universal harmony. (Sheldrake 2011)

Jean Gebser posited: "In magic and mythical man a different kind of 'knowledge' is at work. *He* does not know something; rather, it knows *him,* and, consequently, the circumstances and things affecting him in psychological terms … it is not he, but the 'id', i.e., the 'it' (Freud), the 'unconscious' in him … that knows …" (Gebser 1949/1985).

As we share silent and fertile space, we discover that the intensity of *knowing* and *being* are the same. The feeling of infinity is not only extensively expansive but also deeply intensive.

Community

From a local perspective it begins with each one of us, in communication with ourselves as we unify our body, mind, and spirit and cultivate an advanced consciousness. We commune with others in the group. We find ourselves a part of a fundamental intelligence, a common-unity, a "common unification."

Teacher training necessitates supplying the relevant information. Information can be inspiring but the essence of communication is not reliant on information. Information does not penetrate conditioning. Common unity within an atmosphere of supportive kindness and understanding enables students to trust their perceptions and pass through their impediments. Resistance to receiving is an aspect of conditioned behavior. An individual may let go more easily in the company of others, having the same intention, sharing a light, transcendent prayer free from object and content.

We commune through a prayer of possibility, as we enter the realm of spatial consciousness. We are depth's congregation praying to and from an unknowable place.

We meet within the space of uncluttered essential consciousness. We are connected by the space between us as our personal margins soften. Although each of us has an experience generated by individual perspective, the experience is subject to group energy, space, and consciousness. Body sense and transcendent sense may vary in ascendance for each person at any given moment, but the substrate of consciousness is the same for all involved as they navigate personal depth and understanding.

David Bohm discussed the amount of energy needed to shift the consciousness of mankind and suggested, as yogis and mystics have done for centuries, that deep down there is one consciousness for the whole of mankind:

Chapter 10

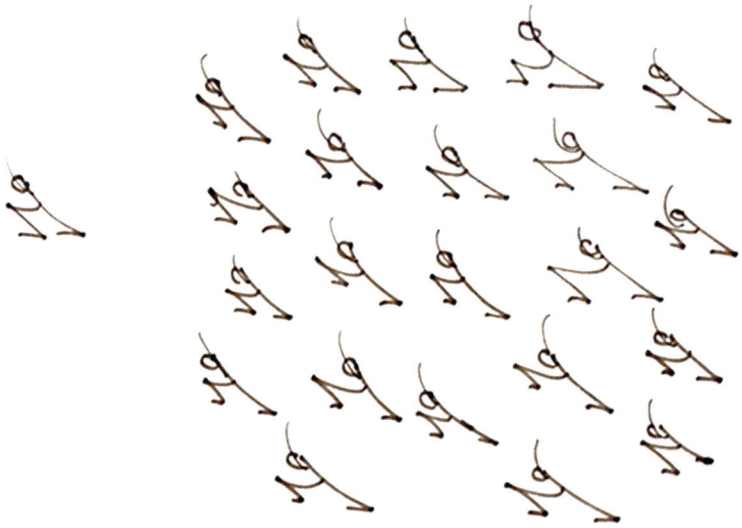

> We share light, transcendent prayer, free from object and content. We commune through a prayer of possibility as we enter the realm of spatial consciousness. We are depth's congregation praying to and from an unknowable place.

It is possible now for a number of individuals who are in close relation ... and can trust each other to establish a one-mind of that whole set of individuals. In other words, that consciousness is one, acting as one. If you had as many as ten people, or a hundred people who could really be that way, they would have a power immensely beyond one ... if ten people can have their part of consciousness all one, that is an energy that begins to spread into the whole. (Bohm in Wilber 1982)

The whole begins with personal totality, a complete sense of self as one is: a place from which we may influence the field around us.

Whatever is or is not out there, it does no harm, and perhaps considerable good, to muse on a benign universal presence, if not a universal or cosmic consciousness then maybe a universal intelligence.

The earth's gravitational field can be seen as a life-producing and sustaining blanket of intelligence arising from a vast beyondness. As our practices plug us into the earth, we tap into a cosmic intelligence, the foundation for human consciousness.

The return of the smile

On occasion, during the height of knowing unknowingness, an impulse to smile arises. It is not a normal smile, but a spontaneous, irrepressible, egoless, intensely satisfying infectious grin, as if one's face may never be the same again, as if the soul celebrates escaping its camouflage. You sense it coming: a dynamic, transformative expression of deep change. It may spread throughout the group!

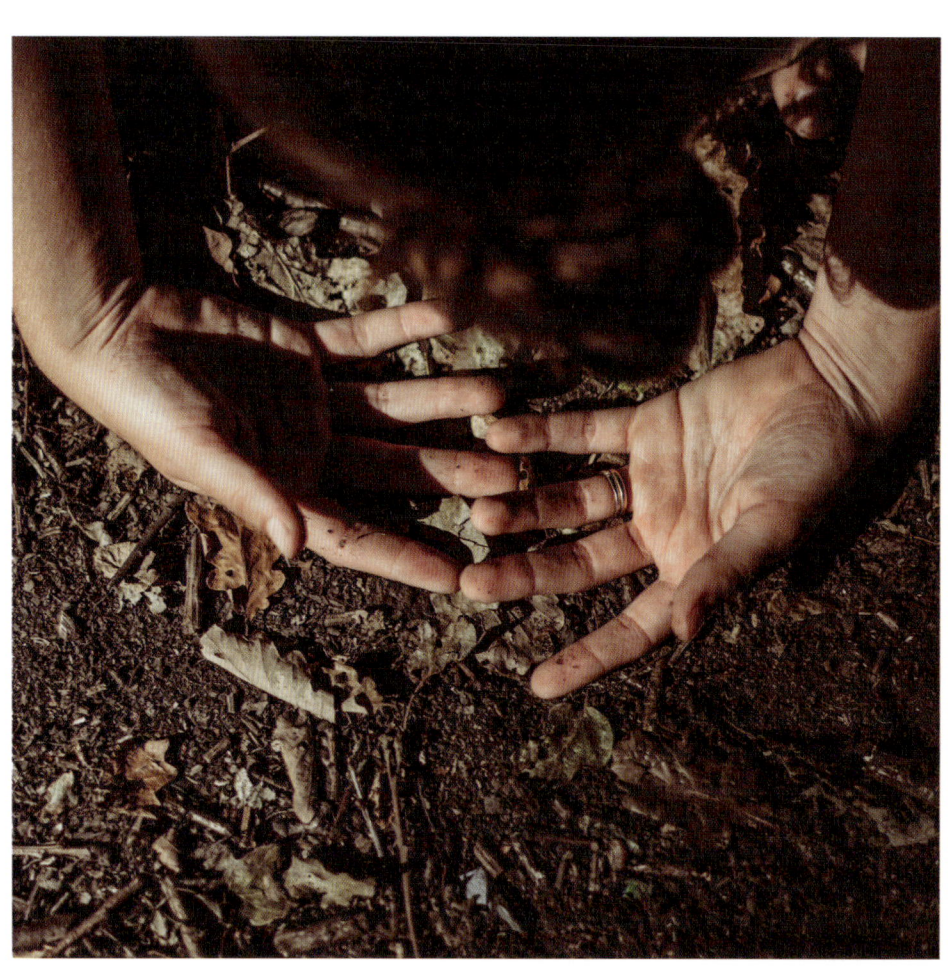

REFERENCES

References

Baker I (2004) The Heart of the World: A Journey to the Last Secret Place. Penguin Press.

Chambers Dictionary of Etymology (2008) Edinburgh: Chambers Harrap Publishers Ltd.

Clay J (1996) R. D. Laing: A Divided Self. London: Hodder and Stoughton.

The Dalai Lama, Cutler HC (1998) The Art of Happiness: A Handbook for Living. London: Hodder and Stoughton.

Damasio A (2000) The Feeling of What Happens: Body and Emotion in the Making of Consciousness. London: Random House.

Desikachar TKV, Krusche H (2014) Freud and Yoga: Two Philosophies of Mind Compared. New York: North Point Press.

Feuerstein G (1974) Wholeness or Transcendence. New York: Larson Publications.

Feuerstein G (1992) Wholeness or Transcendence: Ancient Lessons for the Emerging Global Civilization. New York: Larson Publications.

Feuerstein G (1997) Lucid Waking: Mindfulness and the Spiritual Potential of Humanity. Rochester, Vermont: Inner Traditional International.

Feuerstein G (2003) The Deeper Dimension of Yoga: Theory and Practice. Boston: Shambala Publications.

Fouillée AJE (1887) The language of the emotions. Popular Science Monthly, Volume 31, October 92–126.

Frankl VE (1946/1959) Man's Search for Meaning. UK: Rider, Random House.

Freud S (1921/1959) Group Psychology and the Analysis of the Ego. London: Hogarth Press.

Freud S (1927/1962) The Ego and the Id. London: Hogarth Press.

Gebser J (1949/1985) The Ever-Present Origin. Authorized translation by Noel Barstad with Algis Mickunas. Athens: Ohio University Press.

Goswami A (1995) The Self-Aware Universe: How Consciousness Creates the Material World. New York: Tarcher/Putnam Books.

Guimberteau J-C, Armstrong C (2015) Architecture of Human Living Fascia: The Extracellular Matrix and Cells Revealed through Endoscopy. Edinburgh: Handspring Publishing.

Iyengar BKS (2005) Light on Life: The Yoga Journey to Wholeness, Inner Peace, and Ultimate Freedom. London: Rodale Publishing.

James W (1884) What is an Emotion? Mind os-IX (34) April 188–205.

James W (1902/2018) The Varieties of Religious Experience: A Study in Human Nature. New York: Dover Thrift Editions.

Juhan D (1987) Job's Body: A Handbook for Body Work. Barrytown, NY: Station Hill Press.

REFERENCES *continued*

Kierkegaard S (1844/1980) The Concept of Anxiety: A Simple Psychologically Orienting Deliberation on the Dogmatic Issue of Hereditary Sin. Edited and translated by R Thomte, in collaboration with A Anderson. Chichester, UK: Princeton University Press.

Krishnamurti J (1954/1975) The First and Last Freedom, Krishnamurti Foundation of America. New York: Harper Collins.

Krishnamurti J (1969) Freedom From The Known. Krishnamurti Foundation Trust Ltd.

Laing RD (1960/2010) The Divided Self. London: Penguin Classics.

Laing RD (1982) The Voice of Experience. New York: Pantheon Books, Random House.

Lewis T, Amini F, Lannon R (2000) A General Theory of Love. New York: Vintage Books.

Lipton BH (2008) The Biology of Belief: Unleashing the Power of Consciousness, Matter & Miracles. London: Hay House.

Lowen A (1958) The Language of the Body. Hinesburg: The Alexander Lowen Foundation.

McLynn FJ (1996) Carl Gustav Jung: A Biography. London: Bantam Press.

McTaggart L (2003) The Field. New York: Harper Collins.

Mindell A (1992) Riding the Horse Backwards. Oregon, USA: Lao Tse Press.

Murphy M (1994) The Future of the Body: Explorations into the Future Evolution of Human Nature. New York: Tarcher/Perigee Books.

Odent M (1999) The Scientification of Love. London: Free Association Books Ltd.

Oschman JL (2000) Energy Medicine: The Scientific Basis. London: Churchill Livingstone Elsevier.

Pert CB (1998) Molecules of Emotion: Why You Feel the Way You Feel. London: Simon & Schuster.

Pollan M (2018) How to Change your Mind: The New Science of Psychedelics. UK: Allen Lane.

Sheldrake R (2011) The Presence of the Past: Morphic Resonance and the Habits of Nature. London: Icon Books.

Shorter Oxford English Dictionary (1973). Oxford University Press.

Still AT (1892/1986) The Philosophy and Mechanical Principles of Osteopathy. Kirksville, MO: Osteopathic Enterprise.

Stirk J (2015) The Original Body: Primal Movement for Yoga Teachers. Edinburgh: Handspring Publishing.

Wilber K (Ed.) (1982) The Holographic Paradigm and Other Paradoxes: Exploring the Leading Edge of Science. Boulder, Colorado: Shambala Publications Ltd.

Index

A

Abstruse   130
A General Theory of Love   118
Anchors   15
Archaic consciousness   39
Architecture of Human Living Fascia   68
Attention   47, 113, 155
Attention and awareness   154
Attention and consciousness   158
Authentic   139
Awakening consciousness   13, 30
Awareness   157
Awareness of tension   158

B

Bergson, Henri   127
Body cavities   98
Bohm, David   63, 100
Buddhism   121

C

Cell-free spaces   74
Centers of sensation   97
Community   179–80
Conditioned reactions   161
Confrontation   160
Consciousness   11, 25–30, 35, 36, 37, 38,
    39, 42, 45, 47, 56–57, 62
    archaic   39
    autobiographical self   48
    basic   26
    categories of   54
    dynamic   41
    evolutionary phases of   36
    extended   40
    integral   40–41
    magical   39
    mental   40
    mythical   39
    neural and chemical routes   26
    primitive sensory structures   26
    pure   41
    spatial   40
Consciousness contraction   169
Constructive and obstructive cores   100

Craniosacral Therapy   31
Creative awareness   140
Creative engagement   6
Creativity and conditioning   144
Cyberspace   105

D

Damasio, Antonio   26, 36
Deep body awareness   20
Deep connective tissue   27
Deepening sensation   29–30
Densification   62, 76
Dependency   15–16
Depth   27
Depth of embodiment   28–29
    material depth   27
    nonmaterial depth   27
    unitive awareness   27
Dermatomes   71
Discomfort   9
Dropping down   31
Dynamic consciousness   13, 31, 41, 59

E

Ego   48
    creativity   143
    expansion   52–53
    obstructive and constructive   54
    resistance   53
    sensation   51–52
Emanationism   98
Embodied yoga   25
Embryonic surface tissue   30
Emotional creativity   142
Emotions   95
Enlightenment   11
Essential core   101
Expansion and contraction   114–15
Extended consciousness   40

F

Feuerstein, Georg   41
Fibrils   74
Field of consciousness   89
Fields   83

Fields of influence   83
Fluid creativity   142
Freud's theory of repression   44

G

Gebser, Jean   9
Graphic   166

H

How To Change Your Mind   169

I

Implantation   29
Information   2
Instinct   127
Integral consciousness   40–41
Intellectual creativity   144
Intimacy   116–17
Intuition   127

K

Knowing   21, 100, 166, 168, 178, 179
Knowledge   131

L

Limbic brain   117
Limbic resonance   118
Living tissue   10

M

Magical consciousness   39
Mechanical creativity   141
Memory   42, 128
Mental consciousness   40

INDEX continued

Microvacuolar space 74
Microvacuoles 74
Moments 21
Mystic 112
Mythical consciousness 39

O

Odent, Michel 111
Organic creativity 141
Originality 147

P

Permutations 71
Process 13
Psychoanalysis 55
Pure consciousness 41

Q

Quantum 85
Quantum field theory (QFT) 83
Quantum physics 99, 122, 170

R

Rational consciousness 41

Remote 105
 control 105
 sensing 105
Resonant communication 107
Respiratory creativity 141–42

S

Security 16
Selfhood 45
Selves
 autobiographical self 48
 core self 47–48
 protoself 47
Sensation 27–28, 30, 163
 consciousness 28
 emotion 114
Sensory creativity 140–41
Sentience 64
Shorter Oxford English Dictionary 57
Silence 104
Spatial consciousness 41, 74, 175
Spatial sensations 75, 78
Spiritual creativity 142
Stalling 134
Surface sensation 62

T

Tantra 163
The Biology of Belief 56
The Concept of Anxiety 8
The Crowd: A Study of the Popular Mind 102

The Deeper Dimension of Yoga 74
The Divided Self 35, 43
The Feeling of What Happens 26
The Field 83
The First and Last Freedom 22
The Group Mind 102
The Presence of the Past 85
The Self-Aware Universe 172, 174
Thinking 42
Tissue engagement 30
Transcendence 31
Transcendent 31
Triune brain theory 117

U

Ultimate embodiment 31
Uncalmness 153
Unification 151
 attention 113
Universal sensation 173
Unrefined presence 147

V

Vulnerability 120–21

W

Waiting 142
Wisdom 130